ESR UNVEILED

Understanding the Dynamics of Inflammation

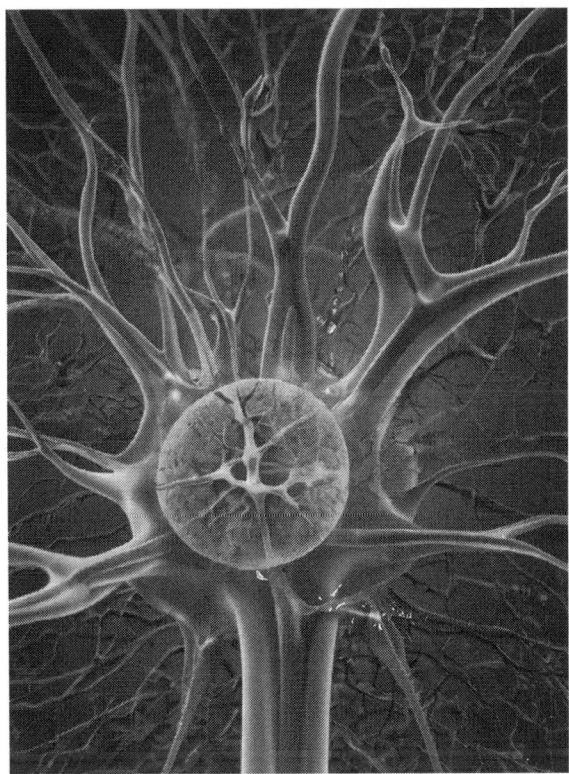

Table of Contents

I. Introduction to Inflammation 2
    A. Definition and basic concepts 4
    B. Historical perspective 5
    C. Importance of inflammation in health and disease 6

II. The Role of Erythrocyte Sedimentation Rate (ESR) 8
    A. Definition and measurement 9
    B. Historical development 10
    C. Clinical significance 12

III. Cellular and Molecular Basis of Inflammation 14
    A. Overview of inflammatory response 16

B. Cellular players: neutrophils, macrophages, lymphocytes, etc. 17

C. Molecular mediators: cytokines, chemokines, prostaglandins, etc. 19

IV: ESR as a Marker of Inflammation 20

    A. Mechanisms underlying ESR elevation in inflammation 21

    B. Relationship between ESR and other inflammatory markers 23

    C. Clinical applications and limitations of ESR measurement 24

V. Understanding Inflammatory Diseases through ESR 26

    A. Inflammatory joint diseases: rheumatoid arthritis, osteoarthritis, etc. 28

    B. Inflammatory bowel diseases: Crohn's disease, ulcerative colitis 29

    C. Infectious diseases: tuberculosis, pneumonia, etc. 30

    D. Autoimmune Diseases: Lupus, Multiple Sclerosis, and Beyond 32

VI. Diagnostic Approach and Interpretation of ESR 33

    A. Interpretation of ESR results in clinical practice 35

    B. Factors affecting ESR measurement 36

    C. Differential diagnosis based on ESR levels 38

VII. Advances in ESR Measurement and Interpretation 39

    A. Modern techniques for ESR measurement 41

    B. Role of ESR kinetics in monitoring disease progression and treatment response 43

    C. Future directions in ESR research.. 44

VIII. Clinical Implications and Future Perspectives 46

    A. ESR-guided management strategies in various diseases 48

    B. Potential role of ESR in personalized medicine 49

    C. Emerging trends in inflammation research and implications for ESR 51

IX. Conclusion 53

I. Introduction to Inflammation

Inflammation: a term both ubiquitous and enigmatic in its nature. At its core, inflammation embodies the body's innate response to injury, infection, or irritation, a fundamental mechanism as ancient as life itself. Yet, despite its primordial significance, the intricacies of inflammation continue to unravel, revealing a complex interplay of cellular, molecular, and systemic dynamics that govern our body's defines and repair mechanisms.

Picture this: a microscopic battlefield, where a legion of cellular soldiers mobilizes in response to an imminent threat. Neutrophils, swift and relentless, surge forward, engulfing foreign invaders with voracious intent. Macrophages, the vigilant sentinels of tissue integrity, stand poised to engulf debris and orchestrate the cleanup effort. Meanwhile, a symphony of molecular signals fills the air, as cytokines, chemokines, and prostaglandins herald the alarm, summoning reinforcements and modulating the inflammatory cascade.

But what prompts this orchestrated symphony of cellular and molecular actors? Enter the erythrocyte sedimentation rate (ESR), a venerable marker of inflammation that has stood the test of time. Originally described by the Swedish physician Robert Favreau's in 1918 and later refined by Favreau's and Westergren in 1921, the ESR represents a simple yet profound reflection of the body's inflammatory state.

Imagine a clear tube filled with blood, left undisturbed on a laboratory bench. Over time, a remarkable phenomenon occurs: the blood gradually separates into distinct layers, with red blood cells settling at the bottom and plasma rising above. This sedimentation process, influenced by various factors including the concentration of acute-phase proteins like fibrinogen, accelerates in the presence of inflammation, leading to an elevated ESR.

But why does inflammation accelerate the sedimentation of red blood cells? The answer lies in the intricate interplay between plasma proteins and the physical properties of blood. Inflammatory stimuli trigger the liver to release acute-phase proteins, such as fibrinogen, into the bloodstream. These proteins interact with red blood cells, causing them to aggregate and form rouleaux, stacked coin-like structures that settle more rapidly due to their increased density.

However, the ESR is not merely a passive bystander in the drama of inflammation; it serves as a sentinel, a harbinger of systemic disturbances that may lurk beneath the surface. Elevated ESR levels may herald the presence of inflammatory conditions ranging from infectious diseases to autoimmune disorders, providing clinicians with a valuable clue in the diagnostic puzzle.

Yet, like any diagnostic tool, the ESR possesses its limitations and nuances. Factors such as age, gender, and certain physiological states can influence ESR values, necessitating a judicious interpretation grounded in clinical context. Moreover, while elevated ESR often correlates with the severity and activity of inflammation, it is not a specific marker for any particular disease, underscoring the importance of a comprehensive diagnostic approach.

As we embark on this journey into the realm of inflammation, let us heed the call of curiosity and inquiry, for within the enigmatic folds of inflammation lie the secrets of health and disease, waiting to be unveiled. Join me as we delve deeper into the labyrinth of inflammation, guided by the steady beacon of the erythrocyte sedimentation rate, towards a greater understanding of the dynamics that shape our physiological landscape.

A. Definition and basic concepts

Inflammation, the cornerstone of the body's defines and repair mechanisms, defies simplistic categorization; it is a multifaceted process with profound implications for health and disease. At its essence, inflammation represents a coordinated response to tissue injury, infection, or irritation, orchestrated by a symphony of cellular and molecular players.

But what precisely constitutes inflammation? To define inflammation is to grasp the essence of physiological chaos and orchestrated harmony that unfolds within our bodies in response to perturbation. Conventionally, inflammation encompasses a constellation of cardinal signs and symptoms: heat, redness, swelling, pain, and loss of function. These outward manifestations, first described by the Roman encyclopaedist Celsus over two millennia ago, serve as tangible manifestations of the underlying inflammatory process.

However, inflammation transcends mere outward appearances; at its core lies a cascade of cellular and molecular events orchestrated with exquisite precision. Picture a bustling metropolis, teeming with activity as cells communicate, migrate, and interact in a choreographed dance of survival and repair. Neutrophils, the foot soldiers of inflammation, rush to the scene, drawn by chemical signals released by injured tissues and activated immune cells. These phagocytic warriors engulf and neutralize invading pathogens, limiting their spread and preventing systemic infection.

But inflammation is not solely a battle against external foes; it is also a delicate balancing act between destruction and regeneration. Macrophages, the scavengers of the immune system, clear away debris and orchestrate tissue repair, laying the foundation for healing and restoration. Meanwhile, a pantheon of molecular mediators, including cytokines, chemokines, and lipid mediators, fine-tune the inflammatory response, modulating its intensity and duration to match the needs of the body.

At its essence, inflammation represents a double-edged sword, capable of both protecting and harming the body depending on its context and magnitude. Acute inflammation, characterized by a rapid onset and resolution, serves as a vital defines mechanism against infectious pathogens and tissue injury. However, when inflammation persists unchecked, it can become chronic, leading to tissue damage, organ dysfunction, and the development of chronic diseases such as arthritis, atherosclerosis, and inflammatory bowel disease.

Yet, despite its central role in health and disease, inflammation remains a complex and enigmatic phenomenon, with many aspects still awaiting elucidation. From the intricacies of immune cell signalling to the interplay between genetic and environmental factors, the study of inflammation continues to yield new insights and therapeutic targets, offering hope for the treatment and prevention of a myriad of human ailments.

As we embark on this journey into the heart of inflammation, let us embrace the complexity and nuance of this fundamental biological process. For within the tangled web of cellular interactions and molecular signals lies the key to unlocking the mysteries of health and disease, guiding us towards a future where inflammation is not merely feared but understood, harnessed, and ultimately mastered for the betterment of humankind.

B. Historical perspective

To understand inflammation is to delve into the annals of medical history, tracing the evolution of our understanding from ancient times to the present day. Indeed, the story of inflammation is as old as medicine itself, intertwined with the rise of civilization and the quest to conquer disease.

The earliest accounts of inflammation can be found in the medical texts of ancient civilizations such as Egypt, Mesopotamia, and India. Ancient healers recognized the cardinal signs of inflammation—heat, redness, swelling, pain—and attributed them to imbalances in bodily humours or the wrath of vengeful gods. Treatments often cantered around rituals, prayers, and herbal remedies, reflecting the mystical and spiritual conceptions of disease prevalent in pre-scientific societies.

It was not until the classical era of Greek and Roman medicine that inflammation began to be studied in a more systematic manner. The Greek physician Hippocrates, often hailed as the father of Western medicine, described inflammation as part of the body's natural response to injury, emphasizing the importance of observation and empirical reasoning in medical practice. His aphorism "First, do no harm" laid the foundation for a more rational and systematic approach to disease.

In the centuries that followed, the concept of inflammation continued to evolve, shaped by the contributions of pioneering scholars and clinicians. The Roman encyclopaedist Celsus provided one of the earliest systematic descriptions of inflammation in his seminal work "De Medicine," distinguishing between acute and chronic forms of the condition. Galen, a towering figure in ancient medicine, further elaborated on the pathophysiology of inflammation, proposing the theory of humoral imbalance and emphasizing the importance of blood and bodily fluids in health and disease.

The Renaissance marked a watershed moment in the history of inflammation, as advances in anatomy, physiology, and microscopy paved the way for a more detailed understanding of the inflammatory process. The pioneering work of anatomists such as Vesalius and Harvey laid bare the intricate structure of the human body, while the invention of the microscope enabled scientists to observe inflammation at the cellular level for the first time.

In the 19th century, the advent of experimental medicine and the rise of pathological anatomy ushered in a new era of scientific inquiry into inflammation. Pathologists such as Rudolf Virchow and Carl Rokitansky meticulously dissected inflamed tissues, cataloguing their findings and laying the groundwork for modern pathology. Meanwhile, researchers such as Louis Pasteur and Robert Koch identified the microbial culprits behind infectious diseases, revolutionizing our understanding of inflammation and paving the way for the development of antimicrobial therapies.

The 20th century witnessed further strides in our understanding of inflammation, fuelled by advances in immunology, biochemistry, and molecular biology. The discovery of cytokines, chemical messengers that regulate the immune response, and the elucidation of signalling pathways involved in inflammation provided new insights into the pathogenesis of inflammatory diseases. Meanwhile, the development of new imaging techniques such as MRI and PET enabled clinicians to visualize inflammation in real-time, revolutionizing diagnosis and treatment.

As we stand on the threshold of the 21st century, the story of inflammation continues to unfold, propelled by the relentless march of scientific progress. From the discovery of novel inflammatory mediators to the development of targeted immunotherapies, the quest to unravel the mysteries of inflammation remains as urgent and relevant as ever. And as we look to the future, let us draw inspiration from the lessons of the past, honouring the legacy of those who came before us and striving to build a world where inflammation is not merely understood but conquered, for the benefit of all mankind.

C. Importance of inflammation in health and disease

Inflammation, often portrayed as the body's double-edged sword, wields profound influence over our health and well-being, shaping our physiological landscape in both health and disease. Far from being a mere reaction to injury or infection, inflammation serves as a sentinel, a guardian of homeostasis, and a key orchestrator of the body's defines and repair mechanisms.

At its core, inflammation represents a finely tuned response to perturbation, whether it be trauma, infection, or autoimmune attack. The immediate goal of inflammation is to eliminate the offending agent, neutralize its effects, and initiate the process of tissue repair. To achieve this end, the body enlists an arsenal of cellular and molecular mediators, ranging from phagocytic leukocytes to cytokines, chemokines, and lipid mediators.

In acute inflammation, the body mounts a rapid and localized response, characterized by the classic signs of heat, redness, swelling, pain, and loss of function. Neutrophils, the first responders of the immune system, rush to the site of injury, where they engulf and neutralize invading pathogens through a process known as phagocytosis. Meanwhile, resident tissue macrophages orchestrate the cleanup effort, clearing away debris and apoptotic cells to pave the way for tissue repair.

Yet, inflammation is far from a static process; it is a dynamic and finely regulated cascade of events, governed by a delicate balance of pro-inflammatory and anti-inflammatory signals. At its peak, inflammation is a necessary and adaptive response, essential for host defines and tissue repair. However, when inflammation persists unchecked, it can become chronic, leading to tissue damage, organ dysfunction, and the development of chronic diseases.

Chronic inflammation lies at the heart of many modern-day maladies, from cardiovascular disease and diabetes to cancer and neurodegenerative disorders. Inflammation contributes to the pathogenesis of these conditions through a variety of mechanisms, including oxidative stress, dysregulated immune responses, and aberrant tissue remodelling. In the case of atherosclerosis, for example, chronic inflammation plays a central role in the initiation and progression of plaque formation, leading to narrowing of the arteries and increased risk of heart attack and stroke.

Moreover, inflammation is not merely a bystander in the disease process; it is often an active participant, perpetuating a vicious cycle of tissue injury and immune activation. In autoimmune diseases such as rheumatoid arthritis and lupus, the immune system mistakenly attacks healthy tissues, leading to chronic inflammation and tissue destruction. Similarly, in neurodegenerative disorders like Alzheimer's disease and Parkinson's disease, inflammation contributes to neuronal injury and loss, exacerbating cognitive decline and motor dysfunction.

Yet, despite its dark side, inflammation also harbours the potential for healing and regeneration. In the right context and under the right circumstances, inflammation can promote tissue repair, stimulate angiogenesis, and facilitate wound healing. Indeed, many of the body's most potent regenerative processes, from muscle repair to bone remodelling, are mediated by inflammation.

As we navigate the complex terrain of inflammation, let us heed the lessons of history and the wisdom of the ages. For within the enigmatic folds of inflammation lie the secrets of health and disease, waiting to be unlocked by the steady hand of scientific inquiry. And as we strive to harness the power of inflammation for the betterment of humankind, let us remember that, like fire, inflammation is a force of nature, capable of both destruction and renewal, depending on how we choose to wield it.

II.   The Role of Erythrocyte Sedimentation Rate (ESR)

Inflammation, a fundamental biological process, is a cornerstone of our body's defines and repair mechanisms. Its significance transcends mere reaction to injury or infection; it embodies a dynamic interplay of cellular and molecular events that profoundly influence our health and well-being.

At its essence, inflammation is a complex response orchestrated by the immune system to restore tissue homeostasis in the face of external or internal challenges. Whether triggered by physical trauma, microbial invasion, or autoimmune dysfunction, the overarching goal of inflammation remains consistent: to eliminate threats, neutralize harmful agents, and promote tissue repair.

In acute inflammation, the body swiftly mobilizes an arsenal of immune cells and signalling molecules to the site of injury or infection. Neutrophils, the body's first line of defines, rapidly infiltrate the affected tissue, engulfing and neutralizing pathogens through phagocytosis. Meanwhile, resident macrophages initiate the cleanup process, clearing away cellular debris and orchestrating the recruitment of additional immune cells to the site of injury.

Crucially, inflammation is not a static process; it is finely regulated and temporally orchestrated. Once the immediate threat has been neutralized, anti-inflammatory signals kick in to resolve the inflammatory response and promote tissue repair. This delicate balance between pro- and anti-inflammatory forces ensures that inflammation serves its protective purpose without causing excessive tissue damage.

However, when inflammation becomes dysregulated or persists beyond its intended duration, it can transition into a chronic state, leading to tissue damage and dysfunction. Chronic inflammation is implicated in the pathogenesis of numerous diseases, ranging from cardiovascular disorders and metabolic syndrome to autoimmune conditions and neurodegenerative disorders.

In cardiovascular disease, for instance, chronic inflammation plays a pivotal role in the development and progression of atherosclerosis, the underlying cause of heart attacks and strokes. Inflammatory processes within the arterial wall promote the formation of plaques, which can rupture and trigger thrombotic events, leading to acute cardiovascular events.

Similarly, in autoimmune diseases such as rheumatoid arthritis and systemic lupus erythematosus, the immune system mistakenly targets healthy tissues, leading to chronic inflammation and tissue destruction. This sustained immune activation can result in joint damage, organ dysfunction, and systemic complications, profoundly impacting the quality of life of affected individuals.

Moreover, emerging evidence suggests that chronic inflammation may contribute to the pathogenesis of age-related diseases, including Alzheimer's disease, Parkinson's disease, and certain cancers. Inflammation within the central nervous system can exacerbate neuronal injury and neurodegeneration, while inflammation in the tumour microenvironment can promote tumour growth, angiogenesis, and metastasis.

Yet, despite its association with disease pathology, inflammation also serves essential functions in tissue repair, regeneration, and immune surveillance. In the context of wound healing, for example, inflammation orchestrates a series of events that culminate in tissue remodelling and scar formation, ensuring the restoration of structural integrity and barrier function.

In conclusion, inflammation is a double-edged sword, capable of both protecting and harming the body depending on its context and duration. By deciphering the intricacies of inflammation, we gain valuable insights into the pathogenesis of disease and identify novel therapeutic targets for intervention. Moreover, by harnessing the regenerative potential of inflammation, we pave the way for innovative approaches to tissue repair and regeneration, offering hope for the prevention and treatment of a wide range of human ailments.

A. Definition and measurement

At the heart of understanding inflammation lies the ability to define and measure this complex biological process. Yet, to confine inflammation within a single definition is to oversimplify its multifaceted nature. In essence, inflammation encompasses a series of dynamic responses orchestrated by the immune system in reaction to tissue injury, infection, or other forms of perturbation. It is not merely a static state but a highly regulated and temporally coordinated cascade of events aimed at restoring tissue homeostasis.

Measurement of inflammation, therefore, becomes a critical endeavour in both clinical and research settings. Among the myriad methods available, one of the oldest and most widely used is the assessment of the erythrocyte sedimentation rate (ESR). This simple yet powerful test provides valuable insights into the inflammatory status of an individual by measuring the rate at which red blood cells settle in a vertical column of blood over a specified period.

The principle behind ESR measurement is elegantly simple: when blood is placed in a vertical tube and allowed to stand undisturbed, red blood cells, being denser than plasma, gradually settle under the influence of gravity. However, in the presence of inflammation, this sedimentation process accelerates due to changes in blood viscosity and plasma protein composition. Specifically, inflammatory stimuli trigger the liver to release acute-phase proteins, such as fibrinogen, into the bloodstream. These proteins interact with red blood cells, causing them to aggregate and form rouleaux, stacked coin-like structures that settle more rapidly than individual cells.

The measurement of ESR, therefore, serves as a surrogate marker of inflammation, reflecting the intensity and duration of the inflammatory response. Elevated ESR levels are commonly observed in a wide range of inflammatory conditions, including infections, autoimmune diseases, and malignancies, making it a valuable tool in clinical diagnosis and monitoring.

However, it is important to recognize that ESR is not a specific marker for any particular disease; rather, it provides a general indication of the presence and severity of inflammation. Moreover, ESR values can be influenced by various factors, including age, gender, and certain physiological states, necessitating careful interpretation in the context of individual patient characteristics.

Despite its limitations, ESR remains a valuable tool in the armamentarium of clinicians and researchers, providing valuable insights into the inflammatory status of patients and guiding diagnostic and therapeutic decisions. Moreover, ongoing advances in technology and methodology continue to refine our ability to measure inflammation, offering new avenues for understanding and treating inflammatory diseases.

In summary, the measurement of inflammation, epitomized by the assessment of ESR, represents a critical component of medical practice and scientific inquiry. By defining and quantifying inflammation, we gain valuable insights into the pathogenesis of disease and identify novel strategies for intervention and management. As our understanding of inflammation continues to evolve, so too will our ability to measure and manipulate this fundamental biological process for the betterment of human health.

B. Historical development

The exploration of inflammation's historical development is akin to embarking on a journey through the annals of medical inquiry, tracing the evolution of our understanding from ancient civilizations to modern science.

This historical odyssey reveals a rich tapestry of discovery, innovation, and paradigm shifts that have shaped our current comprehension of inflammation.

1. **Ancient Roots:**

Inflammation's origins can be traced back to the dawn of civilization, where early healers grappled with the mysteries of illness and injury. Ancient medical texts from civilizations such as Mesopotamia, Egypt, and India provide glimpses into the conceptualization of inflammatory processes. However, these early accounts often intertwined physiological phenomena with mystical and spiritual beliefs, attributing diseases to supernatural forces or imbalances in bodily humours.

2. **Classical Contributions:**

It was in ancient Greece and Rome that the foundations of modern medical thought began to take shape. The Greek physician Hippocrates, often revered as the father of medicine, recognized inflammation as a natural response to injury, emphasizing the importance of observation and rational inquiry in medical practice. His teachings laid the groundwork for a more systematic approach to disease, based on clinical observation and empirical reasoning.

The Roman encyclopaedist Aulus Cornelius Celsus provided one of the earliest systematic descriptions of inflammation in his seminal work "De Medicine," distinguishing between acute and chronic forms of the condition. Meanwhile, Galen, a towering figure in ancient medicine, further elucidated the pathophysiology of inflammation, proposing the theory of humoral imbalance and emphasizing the role of blood and bodily fluids in health and disease.

3. **Renaissance Revelations:**

The Renaissance marked a pivotal period in the history of inflammation, as advances in anatomy, physiology, and microscopy revolutionized our understanding of the human body. Visionary anatomists such as Andreas Vesalius and William Harvey dissected cadavers with unprecedented precision, revealing the intricate architecture of tissues and organs. Meanwhile, the invention of the microscope by pioneers such as Antonie van Leeuwenhoek opened new vistas for scientific inquiry, enabling researchers to observe inflammation at the cellular level for the first time.

4. **The Birth of Pathology:**

The 19th century witnessed the emergence of experimental medicine and the rise of pathological anatomy as disciplines dedicated to unravelling the mysteries of disease. Pathologists such as Rudolf Virchow and Carl Rokitansky meticulously dissected inflamed tissues, cataloguing their findings and laying the groundwork for modern pathology. Meanwhile, the discovery of microbial pathogens by Louis Pasteur and Robert Koch revolutionized our understanding of infectious diseases, linking inflammation to specific microbial agents and paving the way for targeted therapies.

5. The Molecular Revolution:

The 20th century heralded a new era of discovery in inflammation research, as advances in immunology, biochemistry, and molecular biology unravelled the molecular underpinnings of inflammation. The discovery of cytokines, chemical messengers that regulate the immune response, and the elucidation of signalling pathways involved in inflammation provided new insights into the pathogenesis of inflammatory diseases. Meanwhile, the development of new imaging techniques such as MRI and PET enabled clinicians to visualize inflammation in real-time, revolutionizing diagnosis and treatment.

Looking Ahead:

As we stand on the threshold of the 21st century, the story of inflammation continues to unfold, driven by the relentless march of scientific progress. From the discovery of novel inflammatory mediators to the development of targeted immunotherapies, the quest to unravel the mysteries of inflammation remains as urgent and relevant as ever. And as we peer into the future, let us draw inspiration from the lessons of the past, honouring the legacy of those who came before us and striving to build a world where inflammation is not merely understood but conquered, for the benefit of all mankind.

C. Clinical significance

The clinical significance of inflammation extends far beyond its role as a mere physiological response to injury or infection; it is a fundamental determinant of health and disease, shaping the course of countless medical conditions and guiding diagnostic and therapeutic decisions in clinical practice. Understanding the clinical implications of inflammation requires a nuanced appreciation of its diverse manifestations, ranging from acute inflammatory reactions to chronic inflammatory diseases.

1. Acute Inflammation:

Acute inflammation represents the body's rapid and localized response to tissue injury, infection, or other insults. It is characterized by the classic signs of heat, redness, swelling, pain, and loss of function, reflecting the dynamic interplay of cellular and molecular events aimed at restoring tissue homeostasis. Clinically, acute inflammation serves as a diagnostic clue in the evaluation of infectious diseases, trauma, and surgical complications. Elevated inflammatory markers such as C-reactive protein (CRP) and erythrocyte sedimentation rate (ESR) are commonly used in clinical practice to assess the severity and activity of acute inflammatory conditions.

2. **Chronic Inflammatory Diseases:**

Chronic inflammation, by contrast, represents a sustained and dysregulated immune response that can lead to tissue damage, organ dysfunction, and the development of chronic diseases. Chronic inflammatory diseases encompass a broad spectrum of conditions, including autoimmune disorders, metabolic syndrome, neurodegenerative diseases, and certain cancers. Rheumatoid arthritis, for example, is a chronic autoimmune disease characterized by inflammation of the joints, leading to pain, swelling, and progressive joint destruction. Inflammatory bowel diseases (IBD) such as Crohn's disease and ulcerative colitis are chronic inflammatory disorders of the gastrointestinal tract, characterized by abdominal pain, diarrhoea, and mucosal inflammation. In these conditions, the identification of inflammatory biomarkers such as tumour necrosis factor-alpha (TNF-α) and interleukin-6 (IL-6) has revolutionized treatment paradigms, leading to the development of targeted immunotherapies that specifically modulate the inflammatory response.

3. **Cardiovascular Disease:**

Inflammation also plays a central role in the pathogenesis of cardiovascular diseases, including atherosclerosis, myocardial infarction, and stroke. Chronic inflammation within the arterial wall promotes the formation of atherosclerotic plaques, leading to narrowing of the arteries and increased risk of cardiovascular events. Inflammatory biomarkers such as high-sensitivity CRP (his-CRP) and interleukin-6 (IL-6) have emerged as powerful predictors of cardiovascular risk, guiding risk stratification and treatment decisions in clinical practice. Moreover, anti-inflammatory therapies targeting specific inflammatory pathways have shown promise in reducing cardiovascular events, highlighting the therapeutic potential of targeting inflammation in cardiovascular disease management.

4. **Neurodegenerative Diseases:**

In recent years, inflammation has also been implicated in the pathogenesis of neurodegenerative diseases such as Alzheimer's disease, Parkinson's disease, and multiple sclerosis. Chronic inflammation within the central nervous system (CNS) contributes to neuronal injury and neurodegeneration, exacerbating cognitive decline and motor dysfunction. Biomarkers of neuroinflammation, such as microglial activation markers and pro-inflammatory cytokines, hold promise as diagnostic and prognostic indicators in these conditions, guiding treatment decisions and monitoring disease progression.

In summary, inflammation represents a central feature of many medical conditions, influencing their pathogenesis, progression, and response to treatment. By understanding the clinical significance of inflammation and its diverse manifestations, clinicians can better diagnose, manage, and prevent a wide range of inflammatory diseases, ultimately improving patient outcomes and quality of life.

III. Cellular and Molecular Basis of Inflammation

To grasp the intricate workings of inflammation is to delve into the labyrinthine landscape of cellular and molecular interactions that govern this fundamental biological process. At its core, inflammation represents a finely orchestrated symphony of immune cells, signalling molecules, and tissue-resident mediators, each playing a distinct role in orchestrating the body's response to injury, infection, or other insults.

1. **Cellular Players:**

At the forefront of the inflammatory response are the body's immune cells, which act as both sentinels and soldiers in the battle against invading pathogens and tissue damage. Neutrophils, the most abundant type of white blood cell, serve as the first line of defines, rapidly infiltrating inflamed tissues in response to chemical signals released by injured cells and activated immune cells. Armed with potent antimicrobial weapons, neutrophils engulf and neutralize invading pathogens through a process known as phagocytosis, forming the hallmark pus associated with acute inflammation.

Macrophages, the scavengers of the immune system, play a central role in orchestrating the cleanup effort and initiating tissue repair. Derived from circulating monocytes, macrophages patrol the tissues, engulfing and digesting cellular debris, apoptotic cells, and microbial invaders. Moreover, macrophages serve as immune regulators, releasing cytokines, chemokines, and growth factors that modulate the inflammatory response and coordinate tissue remodelling.

Lymphocytes, including T cells, B cells, and natural killer (NK) cells, contribute to both the initiation and resolution of inflammation. T cells, which mature in the thymus, regulate immune responses by recognizing and eliminating infected or aberrant cells. B cells, on the other hand, produce antibodies that neutralize pathogens and facilitate their clearance by other immune cells. NK cells, meanwhile, serve as the body's first line of defines against viral infections and cancer, destroying infected or malignant cells through direct cytotoxicity.

2. **Molecular Mediators:**

At the molecular level, inflammation is governed by a diverse array of signalling molecules, including cytokines, chemokines, prostaglandins, and leukotrienes, each exerting profound effects on immune cell function and tissue homeostasis.

Cytokines, small proteins secreted by immune cells, serve as the primary messengers of inflammation, regulating immune cell activation, proliferation, and differentiation. Pro-inflammatory cytokines such as tumour necrosis factor-alpha (TNF-α), interleukin-1 (IL-1), and interleukin-6 (IL-6) promote inflammation by activating immune cells and inducing the expression of adhesion molecules and inflammatory mediators. Anti-inflammatory cytokines, such as interleukin-10 (IL-10) and transforming growth factor-beta (TGF-β), dampen the inflammatory response and promote tissue repair and resolution.

Chemokines, a subset of cytokines, act as chemoattractant, guiding immune cells to sites of inflammation in response to chemical gradients. By binding to specific receptors on immune cells, chemokines coordinate the recruitment and migration of leukocytes, ensuring their timely arrival at sites of infection or tissue injury.

Prostaglandins and leukotrienes, lipid mediators derived from arachidonic acid, play key roles in inflammation by modulating vascular permeability, leukocyte recruitment, and immune cell activation. Produced by various cell types, including macrophages and mast cells, prostaglandins and leukotrienes amplify and sustain the inflammatory response, contributing to the hallmark signs of inflammation such as redness, swelling, and pain.

3. Cellular and Molecular Interactions:

The orchestration of inflammation involves a complex interplay of cellular and molecular interactions, finely tuned to ensure an effective and controlled response to injury or infection. Upon encountering microbial pathogens or tissue damage, resident immune cells release pro-inflammatory cytokines and chemokines, triggering the activation and recruitment of additional immune cells to the site of inflammation. Neutrophils and monocytes are recruited from the bloodstream to the inflamed tissue, where they engulf pathogens, clear cellular debris, and initiate tissue repair. Meanwhile, adaptive immune responses, mediated by T cells and B cells, provide long-lasting immunity against specific pathogens and contribute to the resolution of inflammation through the production of anti-inflammatory cytokines and regulatory molecules.

In summary, the cellular and molecular basis of inflammation represents a complex and intricately regulated process, governed by a diverse array of immune cells and signalling molecules. By unravelling the molecular mechanisms underlying inflammation, researchers gain valuable insights into the pathogenesis of inflammatory diseases and identify novel targets for therapeutic intervention. Moreover, a deeper understanding of cellular and molecular interactions in inflammation holds promise for the development of personalized approaches to disease management, tailored to the specific needs of individual patients.

A. Overview of inflammatory response

The inflammatory response is a fundamental component of the body's immune system, serving as a protective mechanism against tissue injury, infection, and other insults. It is a complex and highly regulated process involving a cascade of cellular and molecular events aimed at eliminating pathogens, clearing damaged tissues, and promoting tissue repair. Understanding the intricacies of the inflammatory response is essential for elucidating the role of erythrocyte sedimentation rate (ESR) as a marker of inflammation and interpreting its clinical significance.

Initiation of Inflammation:

- Inflammation can be triggered by various stimuli, including microbial pathogens (e.g., bacteria, viruses, fungi), physical trauma, chemical irritants, and autoimmune reactions.
- Recognition of these stimuli by innate immune cells, such as macrophages, dendritic cells, and mast cells, leads to the activation of signalling pathways and the release of pro-inflammatory mediators.

Cellular Events:

- Recruitment of leukocytes, including neutrophils, monocytes, and lymphocytes, to the site of inflammation is a hallmark of the inflammatory response.
- Chemotactic factors, such as cytokines (e.g., interleukin-8) and chemokines, guide leukocytes to the site of injury or infection, where they undergo extravasation from the bloodstream into the affected tissue.

Molecular Mediators:

- Pro-inflammatory cytokines, such as tumour necrosis factor-alpha (TNF-α), interleukin-1 (IL-1), and interleukin-6 (IL-6), play key roles in orchestrating the inflammatory response.
- These cytokines activate endothelial cells, leading to increased vascular permeability and the expression of adhesion molecules that facilitate leukocyte recruitment and extravasation.

Tissue Damage and Repair:

- Inflammatory mediators, including reactive oxygen species (ROS) and proteolytic enzymes, contribute to tissue damage and destruction.
- Simultaneously, anti-inflammatory cytokines (e.g., interleukin-10) and pro-resolving mediators (e.g., lipoxins, resolving) are produced to dampen inflammation and promote tissue repair.

Resolution of Inflammation:

- The inflammatory response is tightly regulated to prevent excessive tissue damage and promote resolution.
- Pro-resolving mediators, such as specialized pro-resolving lipid mediators (SPMs), actively terminate inflammation by inhibiting pro-inflammatory signalling pathways and enhancing the clearance of apoptotic cells and debris.

Systemic Effects:

- In addition to local tissue responses, inflammation can have systemic effects, including fever, leucocytosis, and acute-phase protein synthesis.
- Systemic inflammatory responses may contribute to the pathogenesis of various diseases, including sepsis, autoimmune disorders, and cardiovascular diseases.

Understanding the dynamic interplay of cellular and molecular events underlying the inflammatory response provides insights into the pathophysiology of inflammatory diseases and informs the interpretation of inflammatory markers such as ESR. By elucidating the mechanisms of inflammation, researchers and clinicians can develop targeted therapeutic interventions to modulate the inflammatory response and improve patient outcomes in inflammatory conditions.

B. Cellular players: neutrophils, macrophages, lymphocytes, etc.

Within the intricate tapestry of inflammation, a diverse cast of cellular protagonists plays pivotal roles in orchestrating the body's response to injury, infection, or other insults. From the rapid responders to the architects of tissue repair, each cell type contributes uniquely to the dynamic and finely regulated process of inflammation.

1. **Neutrophils:**

Neutrophils, the most abundant type of white blood cell in the circulation, are the frontline defenders of the innate immune system. These highly specialized cells are equipped with an arsenal of antimicrobial weapons, including phagocytic receptors, antimicrobial peptides, and reactive oxygen species, allowing them to swiftly engulf and neutralize invading pathogens. Neutrophils are recruited to sites of inflammation by chemotactic signals released by injured tissues and activated immune cells, where they form the hallmark pus associated with acute inflammation. Although short-lived, neutrophils play a crucial role in containing microbial infections and initiating the inflammatory cascade.

2. **Macrophages:**

Macrophages, derived from circulating monocytes, are the architects of the immune response, orchestrating the cleanup effort and initiating tissue repair. These versatile cells patrol the tissues, scavenging cellular debris, apoptotic cells, and microbial invaders. Moreover, macrophages serve as immune regulators, releasing cytokines, chemokines, and growth factors that modulate the inflammatory response and coordinate tissue remodelling. Through their phagocytic and immunomodulatory functions, macrophages play a central role in both the initiation and resolution of inflammation, shaping the overall outcome of the inflammatory process.

3. **Lymphocytes:**

Lymphocytes, including T cells, B cells, and natural killer (NK) cells, represent the adaptive arm of the immune system, providing specificity and memory to the immune response. T cells, which mature in the thymus, regulate immune responses by recognizing and eliminating infected or aberrant cells. Helper T cells (CD4+) orchestrate the immune response by secreting cytokines that activate other immune cells, while cytotoxic T cells (CD8+) directly kill infected or cancerous cells. B cells, on the other hand, produce antibodies that neutralize pathogens and facilitate their clearance by other immune cells. Natural killer (NK) cells serve as the body's first line of defines against viral infections and cancer, destroying infected or malignant cells through direct cytotoxicity. Through their diverse effector functions, lymphocytes play critical roles in both the innate and adaptive immune responses, shaping the intensity and duration of inflammation.

4. **Mast Cells:**

Mast cells are tissue-resident immune cells primarily known for their role in allergic reactions and anaphylaxis. However, these enigmatic cells also play important roles in inflammation and host defines. Upon activation by microbial pathogens or environmental triggers, mast cells release a plethora of inflammatory mediators, including histamine, leukotrienes, and cytokines, which promote vasodilation, vascular permeability, and recruitment of immune cells to the site of inflammation. Moreover, mast cells interact with other immune cells and contribute to the regulation of both innate and adaptive immune responses, further highlighting their multifaceted roles in inflammation.

5. **Endothelial Cells:**

Endothelial cells, lining the inner surface of blood vessels, play a crucial role in inflammation by regulating vascular permeability, leukocyte trafficking, and immune cell activation. Upon exposure to inflammatory stimuli, endothelial cells undergo a series of changes, including upregulation of adhesion molecules and chemokine receptors, allowing them to capture circulating leukocytes and promote their extravasation into inflamed tissues. Moreover, endothelial cells release cytokines, growth factors, and vasoactive molecules that modulate the inflammatory response and facilitate tissue repair. Through their interactions with immune cells and blood vessels, endothelial cells serve as gatekeepers of inflammation, coordinating the recruitment and activation of immune cells at sites of tissue injury or infection.

In summary, the cellular players in inflammation represent a diverse array of immune cells and tissue-resident mediators, each contributing uniquely to the dynamic and finely regulated process of inflammation. By unravelling the roles of these cellular protagonists, researchers gain valuable insights into the pathogenesis of inflammatory diseases and identify novel targets for therapeutic intervention, ultimately improving our ability to diagnose, treat, and prevent a wide range of inflammatory conditions.

C. Molecular mediators: cytokines, chemokines, prostaglandins, etc.

In the realm of clinical medicine, the erythrocyte sedimentation rate (ESR) stands as a venerable sentinel, offering invaluable insights into the presence and intensity of inflammation within the body. This simple yet powerful test, based on the principle of erythrocyte aggregation, provides clinicians with a window into the dynamic interplay of cellular and molecular events underlying the inflammatory response.

The ESR, also known as the seed rate, reflects the rate at which erythrocytes settle in a vertical column of blood over a specified period, typically one hour. The principle behind the test is elegantly simple: under normal physiological conditions, red blood cells (erythrocytes) settle slowly in the blood due to their characteristic biconcave shape and negative surface charge, which repels them from each other. However, in the presence of inflammation, changes in blood viscosity and plasma protein composition alter the electrostatic forces between red blood cells, causing them to aggregate and form stacks, or rouleaux, which settle more rapidly.

The process of erythrocyte aggregation is influenced by various factors, including the concentration of plasma proteins, such as fibrinogen and immunoglobulins, which act as molecular bridges between erythrocytes, facilitating their aggregation. Moreover, inflammatory cytokines, such as interleukin-6 (IL-6) and tumour necrosis factor-alpha (TNF-α), promote the production of acute-phase proteins in the liver, including fibrinogen and C-reactive protein (CRP), which further accelerate erythrocyte sedimentation.

Clinically, the ESR serves as a nonspecific marker of inflammation, reflecting the intensity and duration of the inflammatory response rather than providing specific diagnostic information about the underlying cause. Elevated ESR levels are commonly observed in a wide range of inflammatory conditions, including infections, autoimmune diseases, and malignancies, making it a valuable tool in clinical diagnosis and monitoring.

However, it is important to recognize that the ESR is influenced by various factors beyond inflammation, including age, gender, and certain physiological states, such as pregnancy. Moreover, conditions affecting erythrocyte morphology, such as sickle cell disease or spherocytosis, can affect the accuracy of the test results. Therefore, the interpretation of ESR values must be done in the context of the individual patient's clinical presentation and other laboratory findings.

Despite its limitations, the ESR remains a valuable adjunctive tool in the diagnostic workup of inflammatory diseases, providing clinicians with a rapid and cost-effective means of assessing the inflammatory status of patients. Moreover, when used in conjunction with other inflammatory markers, such as CRP and procalcitonin, the ESR can help guide clinical decision-making and monitor response to therapy in various medical conditions.

In summary, the ESR serves as a time-honoured marker of inflammation, reflecting the dynamic changes in blood viscosity and plasma protein composition that accompany the inflammatory response. By providing clinicians with a rapid and accessible means of assessing inflammation, the ESR plays a vital role in the diagnosis and management of a wide range of inflammatory diseases, ultimately improving patient care and outcomes

IV: ESR as a Marker of Inflammation

Erythrocyte sedimentation rate (ESR), a simple yet powerful laboratory test, serves as a cornerstone in the assessment of inflammation and has been utilized for decades in clinical practice as a valuable diagnostic and prognostic tool. Understanding the principles underlying ESR measurement, its clinical significance, and its limitations is essential for healthcare professionals to interpret results accurately and make informed clinical decisions.

1. **Principles of ESR Measurement:**

ESR measurement is based on the principle that erythrocytes (red blood cells) tend to settle more rapidly in a vertical column of blood under the influence of gravity when subjected to an anticoagulant, such as ethylenediaminetetraacetic acid (EDTA). The rate of sedimentation is influenced by various factors, including the concentration and shape of erythrocytes, plasma viscosity, and the presence of plasma proteins. In the presence of inflammation, changes in plasma protein composition, particularly the acute-phase reactant fibrinogen, lead to the formation of rouleaux, stacked coin-like structures of erythrocytes, which settle more rapidly than individual cells. The distance that erythrocytes descend in a specified period, typically one hour, is expressed as the ESR and is measured in millimetres per hour (mm/hr).

2. **Clinical Significance of ESR:**

ESR serves as a nonspecific marker of inflammation, reflecting the intensity and duration of the inflammatory response in the body. Elevated ESR levels are commonly observed in a wide range of inflammatory conditions, including infections, autoimmune diseases, malignancies, and tissue injuries. In acute inflammation, such as bacterial infections or acute trauma, ESR levels typically rise rapidly within hours to days and may reach very high values. Conversely, in chronic inflammatory conditions, such as rheumatoid arthritis or inflammatory bowel disease, ESR levels may be persistently elevated over time, albeit to a lesser extent. Moreover, changes in ESR values over time can provide valuable insights into disease activity, response to treatment, and prognosis, guiding clinical management decisions.

3. **Limitations of ESR:**

Despite its widespread use, ESR has several limitations that must be considered when interpreting results. Firstly, ESR is a nonspecific marker of inflammation and can be influenced by various factors, including age, gender, haematocrit, and certain physiological states, such as pregnancy or menstruation. Moreover, ESR levels may be affected by conditions unrelated to inflammation, such as anaemia, hyperlipidaemia, and chronic renal failure, leading to false-positive or false-negative results. Additionally, ESR is a relatively crude measure of inflammation and lacks the specificity and sensitivity of more advanced laboratory tests, such as C-reactive protein (CRP) or cytokine assays. Therefore, ESR should be interpreted in conjunction with clinical findings and other laboratory tests to obtain a comprehensive assessment of inflammation.

4. **Clinical Applications of ESR:**

Despite its limitations, ESR remains a valuable tool in the armamentarium of clinicians for assessing and monitoring inflammatory conditions. In clinical practice, ESR is commonly used as part of the diagnostic workup for various inflammatory diseases, such as infections, autoimmune disorders, and malignancies. Moreover, serial measurements of ESR over time can provide valuable information about disease activity, response to treatment, and prognosis, guiding therapeutic decisions and patient management strategies. In summary, ESR continues to play a central role in the assessment of inflammation and remains a valuable adjunct to clinical evaluation and other laboratory tests in the diagnosis and management of inflammatory conditions.

In conclusion, ESR serves as a classic marker of inflammation, providing valuable insights into the intensity and duration of the inflammatory response. Despite its limitations, ESR remains a widely used and clinically relevant laboratory test in the assessment of inflammatory diseases. By understanding the principles underlying ESR measurement, its clinical significance, and its limitations, healthcare professionals can effectively utilize this valuable tool to diagnose, monitor, and manage inflammatory conditions, ultimately improving patient care and outcomes.

A. Mechanisms underlying ESR elevation in inflammation

The elevation of erythrocyte sedimentation rate (ESR) in the presence of inflammation reflects a complex interplay of physiological processes orchestrated by the body's response to tissue injury, infection, or other inflammatory stimuli. Understanding the mechanisms underlying ESR elevation provides valuable insights into the dynamic changes that occur within the bloodstream during inflammation.

1. **Plasma Protein Alterations:**

Inflammation triggers a cascade of molecular events that lead to alterations in the composition of plasma proteins, particularly acute-phase proteins synthesized by the liver in response to inflammatory signals. One of the key acute-phase proteins involved in ESR elevation is fibrinogen, a large glycoprotein that plays a central role in blood clotting and inflammatory responses. During inflammation, fibrinogen levels increase in the bloodstream, leading to changes in blood viscosity and the formation of fibrinogen-fibrin complexes that promote erythrocyte aggregation and sedimentation.

2. **Electrostatic Forces:**

Under normal physiological conditions, erythrocytes repel each other due to their negative surface charge, preventing their aggregation and sedimentation in the bloodstream. However, in the presence of inflammation, changes in plasma protein composition and ionic strength alter the electrostatic forces between erythrocytes, allowing them to aggregate and form stacks, or rouleaux, which settle more rapidly. This process of erythrocyte aggregation is facilitated by fibrinogen and other plasma proteins, which act as molecular bridges between erythrocytes, promoting their interaction and sedimentation.

3. **Blood Viscosity:**

Inflammation-induced changes in plasma protein composition and cellular elements, such as leukocytes and platelets, can alter blood viscosity, affecting the rate at which erythrocytes settle in a vertical column of blood. During inflammation, the increased concentration of plasma proteins, particularly fibrinogen, leads to an increase in blood viscosity, promoting erythrocyte aggregation and sedimentation. Moreover, the presence of activated leukocytes and platelets further enhances blood viscosity, contributing to the elevation of ESR in inflammatory conditions.

4. **Haematocrit Changes:**

In addition to alterations in plasma protein composition and blood viscosity, changes in haematocrit, the proportion of blood volume occupied by erythrocytes, can also influence ESR values. Inflammatory stimuli, such as cytokines and growth factors, can stimulate the release of erythropoietin, a hormone that regulates erythropoiesis, leading to an increase in red blood cell production and haematocrit levels. Elevated haematocrit levels can promote erythrocyte aggregation and sedimentation, further contributing to the elevation of ESR in inflammation.

5. **Other Factors:**

Several other factors can affect ESR values in inflammatory conditions, including red blood cell morphology, temperature, and ph. Conditions affecting erythrocyte morphology, such as sickle cell disease or spherocytosis, can affect the rate of erythrocyte aggregation and sedimentation, leading to inaccurate ESR measurements. Moreover, changes in temperature and pH can alter the electrostatic forces between erythrocytes, influencing their aggregation and sedimentation rates.

In summary, the elevation of ESR in inflammation reflects a complex interplay of physiological processes, including alterations in plasma protein composition, blood viscosity, haematocrit levels, and erythrocyte morphology. By understanding the mechanisms underlying ESR elevation, clinicians can better interpret ESR values in the context of inflammatory diseases, improving diagnostic accuracy and patient care.

B. Relationship between ESR and other inflammatory markers

In the intricate landscape of inflammation assessment, the erythrocyte sedimentation rate (ESR) stands as a cornerstone alongside a multitude of other inflammatory markers. Understanding the relationship between ESR and these markers provides crucial insights into the diverse facets of the inflammatory response, guiding diagnostic decisions and therapeutic interventions in clinical practice.

C-Reactive Protein (CRP):

C-reactive protein (CRP), another key acute-phase protein, is synthesized by the liver in response to inflammatory stimuli, particularly interleukin-6 (IL-6). Like ESR, CRP levels increase in the presence of inflammation, making it a valuable marker for assessing systemic inflammation and infection. While both ESR and CRP reflect the intensity of the inflammatory response, they differ in their kinetics and sensitivity to certain inflammatory conditions. CRP typically rises more rapidly in response to acute inflammation and returns to baseline levels more quickly than ESR. However, in chronic inflammatory conditions, such as rheumatoid arthritis or inflammatory bowel disease, CRP and ESR levels may be discordant, highlighting the importance of using multiple inflammatory markers to assess disease activity and response to treatment.

White Blood Cell Count (WBC):

White blood cell count (WBC), a measure of the total number of leukocytes circulating in the bloodstream, is another commonly used marker of inflammation. During inflammation, leukocytes, including neutrophils, lymphocytes, and monocytes, are recruited to sites of infection or tissue injury, leading to an increase in WBC count. While ESR reflects the dynamics of erythrocyte aggregation and sedimentation, WBC count provides information about the cellular components of the inflammatory response. Elevated WBC count, in conjunction with elevated ESR, suggests a more robust inflammatory response and may indicate the presence of bacterial infection or other serious inflammatory conditions.

Procalcitonin (PCT):

Procalcitonin (PCT) is a precursor peptide of calcitonin that is released into the bloodstream in response to bacterial infection or sepsis. Unlike ESR and CRP, which are nonspecific markers of inflammation, PCT is considered a more specific marker of bacterial infection and sepsis. While ESR and CRP may be elevated in a wide range of inflammatory conditions, including viral infections and autoimmune diseases, PCT levels typically remain within normal limits in these conditions. Therefore, combining ESR with PCT can help differentiate between infectious and non-infectious causes of inflammation, aiding in the diagnostic workup and management of patients with suspected infections.

Interleukins (ILs):

Interleukins (ILs) are a family of cytokines that play key roles in regulating the immune response and inflammation. IL-6, in particular, is a potent inducer of acute-phase proteins, including CRP, and is closely associated with the inflammatory cascade. Measurement of IL-6 levels provides valuable insights into the intensity and duration of the inflammatory response and may help guide treatment decisions in inflammatory diseases. Similarly, other pro-inflammatory cytokines, such as tumour necrosis factor-alpha (TNF-α) and interleukin-1 (IL-1), are also implicated in the pathogenesis of inflammatory diseases and can serve as useful markers of disease activity and response to therapy.

Imaging Studies:

In addition to laboratory markers, imaging studies, such as magnetic resonance imaging (MRI), computed tomography (CT), and positron emission tomography (PET), play a crucial role in assessing inflammation and disease activity in various organs and tissues. These imaging modalities provide visual evidence of inflammation, allowing clinicians to localize inflammatory lesions, assess their extent and severity, and monitor response to treatment. When used in conjunction with laboratory markers, imaging studies provide a comprehensive evaluation of inflammatory diseases, facilitating accurate diagnosis and targeted therapy.

In summary, the relationship between ESR and other inflammatory markers provides valuable insights into the dynamic and multifaceted nature of the inflammatory response. By integrating multiple inflammatory markers, clinicians can obtain a more comprehensive assessment of disease activity, guide diagnostic decisions, and tailor treatment strategies to individual patients, ultimately improving outcomes in inflammatory diseases.

C. Clinical applications and limitations of ESR measurement

The measurement of erythrocyte sedimentation rate (ESR) has long served as a cornerstone in the assessment of inflammation and has found widespread clinical application across various medical specialties. However, like any diagnostic test, ESR has both strengths and limitations that must be carefully considered in clinical practice.

Clinical Applications:

1. Screening and Diagnosis:

ESR is frequently used as a screening tool to assess the presence and severity of inflammation in patients presenting with nonspecific symptoms such as fever, fatigue, and malaise. Elevated ESR levels can provide valuable diagnostic clues and guide further evaluation to identify the underlying cause of inflammation, such as infection, autoimmune disease, or malignancy. In combination with clinical history, physical examination, and other laboratory tests, ESR measurement helps clinicians formulate differential diagnoses and prioritize diagnostic investigations.

2. Monitoring Disease Activity:

In chronic inflammatory conditions, such as rheumatoid arthritis, systemic lupus erythematosus, and inflammatory bowel disease, ESR serves as a marker of disease activity and response to therapy. Serial measurements of ESR over time can track changes in inflammatory burden, guiding treatment decisions and monitoring disease progression. A reduction in ESR levels following initiation of treatment may indicate a favourable response, whereas persistently elevated ESR levels may suggest ongoing disease activity or treatment resistance, prompting reassessment and adjustment of therapy.

3. Prognostication:

ESR has prognostic value in certain inflammatory diseases, providing insights into disease severity, prognosis, and risk of complications. In conditions such as giant cell arteritis and polymyalgia rheumatica, elevated ESR levels are associated with an increased risk of vascular complications, such as stroke and vision loss, highlighting the importance of early detection and aggressive management. Similarly, in infectious diseases such as sepsis and pneumonia, elevated ESR levels may indicate an increased risk of morbidity and mortality, prompting closer monitoring and aggressive supportive care.

Limitations:

1. No specificity:

One of the primary limitations of ESR is its lack of specificity, as elevated levels can be observed in a wide range of inflammatory and non-inflammatory conditions. Various factors, including age, gender, pregnancy, anaemia, and certain medications, can influence ESR values, leading to false-positive or false-negative results. Therefore,

ESR should be interpreted in the context of the patient's clinical presentation, medical history, and other laboratory findings to avoid misdiagnosis or unnecessary interventions.

2. **Lag Time:**

ESR is a relatively nonspecific marker of inflammation with a delayed response time, reflecting changes in the acute-phase protein concentration rather than the underlying inflammatory process itself. As a result, ESR may not accurately reflect acute changes in disease activity or response to therapy, particularly in rapidly evolving clinical scenarios. Other inflammatory markers, such as C-reactive protein (CRP) and procalcitonin, may provide more rapid and dynamic assessments of inflammation and guide more timely clinical decisions.

3. **Interlaboratory Variability:**

ESR measurements can vary between different laboratory methods and instrumentation platforms, leading to inconsistencies in results and complicating the interpretation of findings. Standardization of ESR measurement techniques and reference ranges is essential to ensure consistency and comparability across different healthcare settings. Moreover, regular quality control measures and proficiency testing are necessary to maintain the accuracy and reliability of ESR measurements over time.

In summary, while ESR remains a valuable tool in the assessment of inflammation, its clinical utility is tempered by its no specificity, delayed response time, and potential for interlaboratory variability. Clinicians should use ESR judiciously, considering its strengths and limitations in the context of the individual patient's clinical presentation and medical history. Integration of ESR measurement with other inflammatory markers and clinical parameters enhances diagnostic accuracy and improves patient care, ultimately leading to better outcomes for patients with inflammatory diseases.

V. Understanding Inflammatory Diseases through ESR

In the realm of medicine, the erythrocyte sedimentation rate (ESR) serves as a diagnostic beacon, illuminating the pathophysiological landscape of inflammatory diseases and guiding clinicians in their quest to unravel the mysteries of these complex conditions. By examining the dynamic changes in ESR levels, clinicians gain valuable insights into the underlying inflammatory processes, disease activity, and response to therapy, ultimately improving the diagnosis, management, and prognosis of inflammatory diseases.

Diagnostic Insights:

ESR plays a pivotal role in the diagnosis of inflammatory diseases, providing clinicians with a rapid and accessible means of assessing the presence and severity of inflammation. Elevated ESR levels serve as a red flag, alerting clinicians to the possibility of underlying inflammatory conditions such as infection, autoimmune disease, or malignancy. In combination with clinical history, physical examination, and other laboratory tests, ESR measurement helps clinicians formulate differential diagnoses and prioritize diagnostic investigations, leading to timely and accurate diagnosis.

Disease Activity Monitoring:

In chronic inflammatory diseases, such as rheumatoid arthritis, systemic lupus erythematosus, and inflammatory bowel disease, ESR serves as a marker of disease activity and response to therapy. Serial measurements of ESR over time allow clinicians to track changes in inflammatory burden, guiding treatment decisions and monitoring disease progression. A reduction in ESR levels following initiation of treatment may indicate a favourable response, whereas persistently elevated ESR levels may suggest ongoing disease activity or treatment resistance, prompting reassessment and adjustment of therapy.

Prognostic Indicators:

ESR has prognostic value in certain inflammatory diseases, providing insights into disease severity, prognosis, and risk of complications. In conditions such as giant cell arteritis and polymyalgia rheumatica, elevated ESR levels are associated with an increased risk of vascular complications, such as stroke and vision loss, highlighting the importance of early detection and aggressive management. Similarly, in infectious diseases such as sepsis and pneumonia, elevated ESR levels may indicate an increased risk of morbidity and mortality, prompting closer monitoring and aggressive supportive care.

Therapeutic Monitoring:

ESR serves as a valuable tool in monitoring response to therapy and guiding treatment decisions in inflammatory diseases. Serial measurements of ESR allow clinicians to assess the effectiveness of pharmacological interventions, such as anti-inflammatory agents and immunomodulatory therapies, and adjust treatment regimens accordingly. A decrease in ESR levels following initiation of therapy may indicate a positive response, whereas persistently elevated ESR levels may signal treatment failure or the need for alternative therapeutic strategies.

Research and Clinical Trials:

ESR is widely used as an outcome measure in clinical research and therapeutic trials evaluating new treatments for inflammatory diseases. Changes in ESR levels are often used as surrogate endpoints to assess treatment efficacy and safety, providing valuable insights into the clinical benefits and risks of novel therapeutic interventions. Moreover, ESR measurements are incorporated into disease activity indices and scoring systems used in clinical trials to standardize outcome assessments and facilitate comparisons between treatment arms.

In summary, ESR serves as a powerful tool in understanding inflammatory diseases, providing clinicians with valuable insights into disease pathogenesis, activity, and response to therapy. By integrating ESR measurement into clinical practice, clinicians can improve diagnostic accuracy, optimize treatment strategies, and enhance patient outcomes in inflammatory diseases.

A. Inflammatory joint diseases: rheumatoid arthritis, osteoarthritis, etc.

Inflammatory joint diseases encompass a spectrum of conditions characterized by inflammation of the joints, leading to pain, swelling, stiffness, and impaired joint function. Among the most prominent inflammatory joint diseases are rheumatoid arthritis (RA) and osteoarthritis (OA), each with distinct pathophysiological mechanisms, clinical presentations, and management approaches.

1. Rheumatoid Arthritis (RA):

Rheumatoid arthritis is a chronic autoimmune disease characterized by inflammation of the synovial lining of the joints, leading to joint destruction and systemic complications. The pathogenesis of RA involves a dysregulated immune response, with activation of auto-reactive T cells and B cells, production of autoantibodies such as rheumatoid factor (RF) and anti-cyclic citrullinated peptide (anti-CCP), and release of pro-inflammatory cytokines, particularly tumour necrosis factor-alpha (TNF-α) and interleukin-6 (IL-6). These inflammatory mediators drive synovial inflammation, pannus formation, and cartilage destruction, ultimately leading to erosive changes and joint deformities. Clinically, RA typically presents with symmetric polyarthritis affecting the small joints of the hands and feet, with morning stiffness lasting more than 30 minutes.

Extra-articular manifestations, such as rheumatoid nodules, vasculitis, and pulmonary involvement, may also occur. Management of RA involves a multidisciplinary approach, including pharmacological interventions (e.g., disease-modifying anti-rheumatic drugs, biologic agents), physical therapy, and lifestyle modifications, aimed at controlling inflammation, preserving joint function, and improving quality of life.

2. Osteoarthritis (OA):

Osteoarthritis is the most common form of arthritis, characterized by progressive degeneration of the articular cartilage, synovial inflammation, and bony changes within the joints. While traditionally considered a non-inflammatory disease, emerging evidence suggests that low-grade inflammation plays a contributory role in the pathogenesis of OA. Factors such as mechanical stress, aging, obesity, and genetic predisposition contribute to cartilage breakdown and synovial inflammation, leading to joint pain and functional impairment. Inflammatory mediators, including cytokines such as interleukin-1 (IL-1) and tumour necrosis factor-alpha

(TNF-α), are implicated in cartilage degradation, synovitis, and pain sensitization in OA. Clinically, OA typically presents with joint pain, stiffness, and limited range of motion, often affecting weight-bearing joints such as the knees, hips, and spine. Management of OA focuses on symptom relief, functional preservation, and improving quality of life through a combination of non-pharmacological interventions (e.g., exercise, weight management) and pharmacological therapies (e.g., analgesics, non-steroidal anti-inflammatory drugs).

3. **Other Inflammatory Joint Diseases:**

In addition to RA and OA, several other inflammatory joint diseases exist, each with unique clinical features, etiologist, and management strategies. These include:

1. **Psoriatic arthritis:** A chronic inflammatory arthritis associated with psoriasis, characterized by asymmetric oligoarthritic, enthesitis, dactylitis, and nail changes.
2. **Ankylosing spondylitis:** A chronic inflammatory disease primarily affecting the sacroiliac joints and spine, leading to spinal fusion, pain, and stiffness.
3. **Reactive arthritis:** A form of arthritis that develops in response to an infection, typically affecting the joints, eyes, skin, and genitourinary tract.
4. **Juvenile idiopathic arthritis:** A group of chronic inflammatory arthropathies that begin in childhood and are characterized by joint inflammation, stiffness, and systemic features.

In summary, inflammatory joint diseases such as rheumatoid arthritis and osteoarthritis represent significant burdens on individuals and healthcare systems worldwide. Understanding the pathophysiology, clinical manifestations, and management principles of these conditions is essential for optimizing patient care and improving outcomes for individuals affected by these debilitating diseases.

B. Inflammatory bowel diseases: Crohn's disease, ulcerative colitis

Inflammatory bowel diseases (IBD) comprise a group of chronic inflammatory disorders of the gastrointestinal tract, most notably Crohn's disease and ulcerative colitis. These conditions are characterized by recurrent inflammation of the intestines, leading to a range of symptoms, including abdominal pain, diarrhoea, rectal bleeding, weight loss, and fatigue. Understanding the nuances of Crohn's disease and ulcerative colitis is crucial for proper diagnosis, management, and improving the quality of life for affected individuals.

1. **Crohn's Disease:**

Crohn's disease is a chronic inflammatory condition that can affect any part of the gastrointestinal tract, from the mouth to the anus. It is characterized by transmural inflammation, meaning inflammation extends through the entire thickness of the intestinal wall. The exact aetiology of Crohn's disease remains unclear, but it is thought to involve a dysregulated immune response triggered by environmental factors in genetically susceptible individuals. Immune cells infiltrate the intestinal mucosa, leading to the release of pro-inflammatory cytokines, including tumour necrosis factor-alpha (TNF-α), interleukin-6 (IL-6), and interleukin-12 (IL-12), which perpetuate inflammation and tissue damage. Clinically, Crohn's disease can present with a variety of symptoms, including abdominal pain, diarrhoea (which may be bloody), fatigue, weight loss, and extraintestinal manifestations such as arthritis, skin lesions, and ocular inflammation.

The disease course can be highly variable, with periods of remission alternating with flare-ups of active disease. Management of Crohn's disease involves a multidisciplinary approach, including pharmacological therapies (e.g., corticosteroids, immunomodulators, biologic agents), nutritional support, and surgical intervention in cases of complications or refractory disease.

2. **Ulcerative Colitis:**

Ulcerative colitis is a chronic inflammatory disorder that primarily affects the colon and rectum. Unlike Crohn's disease, which can involve any part of the gastrointestinal tract, ulcerative colitis is limited to the mucosal layer of the colon and rectum. The exact aetiology of ulcerative colitis is unknown, but it is believed to result from an abnormal immune response to commensal gut bacteria in genetically predisposed individuals. Inflammation typically begins in the rectum and may extend proximally in a continuous fashion, leading to diffuse mucosal ulceration and inflammation. Pro-inflammatory cytokines, including interleukin-1 (IL-1), interleukin-6 (IL-6), and tumour necrosis factor-alpha (TNF-α), drive the inflammatory process and contribute to tissue damage. Clinically, ulcerative colitis presents with symptoms such as bloody diarrhoea, abdominal pain, urgency, tenesmus, and rectal bleeding. Extra-intestinal manifestations, such as arthritis, uveitis, and skin lesions, may also occur. Management of ulcerative colitis involves pharmacological therapies (e.g., amino salicylates, corticosteroids, immunomodulators, biologic agents), dietary modifications, and surgical options (e.g., colectomy) in severe or refractory cases.

Both Crohn's disease and ulcerative colitis are associated with an increased risk of complications, including intestinal strictures, fistulas, abscesses, and colorectal cancer. Long-term management focuses on controlling inflammation, minimizing symptoms, preventing complications, and improving quality of life. Regular monitoring of disease activity through clinical assessment, laboratory tests (including inflammatory markers such as C-reactive protein and erythrocyte sedimentation rate), endoscopic evaluation, and imaging studies is essential for optimizing treatment and ensuring favourable outcomes for individuals with IBD. Additionally, patient education, psychosocial support, and involvement in shared decision-making are integral components of comprehensive IBD care.

C. Infectious diseases: tuberculosis, pneumonia, etc.

Infectious diseases encompass a broad spectrum of illnesses caused by pathogenic microorganisms such as bacteria, viruses, fungi, and parasites. Among the most prevalent and clinically significant infectious diseases are tuberculosis (TB) and pneumonia, each presenting unique challenges in diagnosis, treatment, and prevention.

1. **Tuberculosis (TB):**

Tuberculosis is a bacterial infection caused by Mycobacterium tuberculosis, a slow-growing acid-fast bacillus that primarily affects the lungs but can also involve other organs such as the lymph nodes, bones, and central nervous system. TB is transmitted through the inhalation of respiratory droplets containing the bacteria, typically from an infected individual with active pulmonary TB. Upon inhalation, M. tuberculosis infects alveolar macrophages and replicates within these cells, leading to the formation of granulomas, which are hallmark lesions of TB. Clinically, TB can present with a wide range of symptoms, including cough, fever, night sweats, weight loss, fatigue, and haemoptysis.

Diagnosis of TB relies on a combination of clinical evaluation, imaging studies (such as chest X-ray or computed tomography), microbiological testing (including sputum smear microscopy, culture, and nucleic acid amplification tests), and tuberculin skin testing or interferon-gamma release assays. Treatment of TB involves a multi-drug regimen, typically including isoniazid, revamping, pyrazinamide, and ethambutol, administered for several months to eradicate the bacteria and prevent the development of drug resistance. Directly observed therapy (DOT) and adherence support are essential components of TB treatment to ensure treatment completion and minimize the risk of treatment failure or relapse.

2. **Pneumonia:**

Pneumonia is an acute respiratory infection characterized by inflammation of the lung parenchyma, typically caused by bacterial, viral, fungal, or atypical pathogens. Streptococcus pneumoniae, Haemophilus influenzae, and Mycoplasma pneumoniae are among the most common causative agents of community-acquired pneumonia (CAP), whereas healthcare-associated pneumonia (HCAP) and hospital-acquired pneumonia (HAP) may be caused by a broader range of pathogens, including multidrug-resistant bacteria. Pneumonia is often classified based on clinical presentation (e.g., typical vs. atypical pneumonia), radiographic findings (e.g., lobar vs. interstitial pneumonia), and aetiology (e.g., bacterial vs. viral pneumonia).

Clinically, pneumonia can present with symptoms such as fever, cough, dyspnoea, chest pain, sputum production, and systemic manifestations such as confusion and sepsis. Diagnosis of pneumonia involves a combination of clinical evaluation, chest imaging (such as chest X-ray or computed tomography), and microbiological testing (including sputum culture, blood culture, and urinary antigen testing). Empirical antibiotic therapy is initiated promptly based on the severity of illness, risk factors for specific pathogens, and local antibiotic resistance patterns. Treatment of pneumonia may involve outpatient oral antibiotics for mild cases of CAP or intravenous antibiotics for severe cases requiring hospitalization. Supportive care measures, including oxygen therapy, hydration, and respiratory support, are essential components of pneumonia management to optimize patient outcomes and prevent complications such as respiratory failure and septic shock.

In summary, tuberculosis and pneumonia are among the most prevalent and clinically significant infectious diseases worldwide, posing considerable challenges to public health and healthcare systems. Early recognition, prompt diagnosis, and timely initiation of appropriate treatment are essential for controlling the spread of these infections, preventing complications, and improving patient outcomes. Additionally, comprehensive strategies for TB and pneumonia prevention, including vaccination, infection control measures, and antimicrobial stewardship, are crucial for reducing the burden of these infectious diseases and achieving global health goals.

D. Autoimmune Diseases: Lupus, Multiple Sclerosis, and Beyond

Autoimmune diseases represent a broad category of disorders in which the immune system mistakenly attacks the body's own tissues, leading to chronic inflammation, tissue damage, and dysfunction. Among the myriad autoimmune conditions, systemic lupus erythematosus (SLE) and multiple sclerosis (MS) stand out as prototypical examples, each with unique pathophysiological mechanisms, clinical manifestations, and management challenges.

1. **Systemic Lupus Erythematosus (SLE):**

Systemic lupus erythematosus is a complex autoimmune disease characterized by multi-system involvement and a broad spectrum of clinical manifestations. The underlying aetiology of SLE is multifactorial, involving genetic predisposition, environmental triggers, hormonal factors, and dysregulated immune responses. In SLE, the immune system produces autoantibodies against nuclear antigens, such as double-stranded DNA (dsDNA), nucleosomes, and ribonucleoproteins, leading to immune complex formation and deposition in various tissues.

This triggers inflammation, tissue injury, and the release of pro-inflammatory cytokines, such as interleukin-6 (IL-6) and tumour necrosis factor-alpha (TNF-α). Clinically, SLE can affect virtually any organ system, with common manifestations including arthritis, skin rashes (e.g., malar rash, discoid rash), renal involvement (e.g., lupus nephritis), hematologic abnormalities (e.g., anaemia, thrombocytopenia), and neuropsychiatric symptoms (e.g., cognitive dysfunction, seizures). The disease course is often characterized by periods of remission and flares, with variable patterns of organ involvement and severity. Management of SLE requires a multidisciplinary approach, including pharmacological therapies (e.g., corticosteroids, antimalarials, immunosuppressants), lifestyle modifications, and close monitoring for disease activity and complications.

2. **Multiple Sclerosis (MS):**

Multiple sclerosis is a chronic inflammatory demyelinating disease of the central nervous system (CNS), characterized by immune-mediated damage to myelin and axons. The exact aetiology of MS remains incompletely understood but is thought to involve genetic susceptibility, environmental triggers (e.g., viral infections), and dysregulated immune responses. In MS, activated T cells and B cells cross the blood-brain barrier and initiate an inflammatory cascade, leading to demyelination, axonal injury, and neurodegeneration. The release of pro-inflammatory cytokines, such as interferon-gamma (IFN-γ) and interleukin-17 (IL-17), further amplifies the inflammatory response and contributes to tissue damage. Clinically, MS can present with a wide range of symptoms, including sensory disturbances, motor weakness, visual impairment, fatigue, and cognitive dysfunction. The disease course can vary widely, with relapsing-remitting, primary progressive, and secondary progressive phenotypes. Management of MS involves disease-modifying therapies (e.g., interferon beta, monoclonal antibodies), symptomatic treatments (e.g., corticosteroids, muscle relaxants), and rehabilitation strategies to optimize function and quality of life.

3. **Other Autoimmune Diseases:**

Beyond SLE and MS, autoimmune diseases encompass a diverse array of conditions affecting virtually every organ system, including rheumatoid arthritis, type 1 diabetes, autoimmune thyroid diseases (e.g., Graves' disease, Hashimoto's thyroiditis), inflammatory bowel diseases (e.g., Crohn's disease, ulcerative colitis), and autoimmune skin disorders (e.g., psoriasis, pemphigus). Each autoimmune disease has its unique pathogenesis, clinical features, and management considerations, but all share a common theme of immune dysregulation and tissue-specific autoimmunity. Management of autoimmune diseases typically involves a combination of immunosuppressive therapies, anti-inflammatory agents, and targeted biologic agents, aimed at suppressing aberrant immune responses, reducing inflammation, and preserving organ function.

In summary, autoimmune diseases represent a diverse group of disorders characterized by dysregulated immune responses against self-tissues. Understanding the underlying mechanisms, clinical manifestations, and therapeutic options for autoimmune diseases is essential for providing optimal care and improving outcomes for affected individuals. A multidisciplinary approach, including collaboration between rheumatologists, neurologists, immunologists, and other specialists, is often necessary to address the complex needs of patients with autoimmune diseases and to tailor treatment strategies to individual patient characteristics and disease manifestations.

VI. Diagnostic Approach and Interpretation of ESR

The inflammatory response is a fundamental component of the body's immune system, serving as a protective mechanism against tissue injury, infection, and other insults. It is a complex and highly regulated process involving a cascade of cellular and molecular events aimed at eliminating pathogens, clearing damaged tissues, and promoting tissue repair. Understanding the intricacies of the inflammatory response is essential for elucidating the role of erythrocyte sedimentation rate (ESR) as a marker of inflammation and interpreting its clinical significance.

1. Initiation of Inflammation:
    - Inflammation can be triggered by various stimuli, including microbial pathogens (e.g., bacteria, viruses, fungi), physical trauma, chemical irritants, and autoimmune reactions.

- Recognition of these stimuli by innate immune cells, such as macrophages, dendritic cells, and mast cells, leads to the activation of signalling pathways and the release of pro-inflammatory mediators.

2. Cellular Events:

    - Recruitment of leukocytes, including neutrophils, monocytes, and lymphocytes, to the site of inflammation is a hallmark of the inflammatory response.
    - Chemotactic factors, such as cytokines (e.g., interleukin-8) and chemokines, guide leukocytes to the site of injury or infection, where they undergo extravasation from the bloodstream into the affected tissue.

3. Molecular Mediators:

    - Pro-inflammatory cytokines, such as tumour necrosis factor-alpha (TNF-α), interleukin-1 (IL-1), and interleukin-6 (IL-6), play key roles in orchestrating the inflammatory response.
    - These cytokines activate endothelial cells, leading to increased vascular permeability and the expression of adhesion molecules that facilitate leukocyte recruitment and extravasation.

4. Tissue Damage and Repair:

    - Inflammatory mediators, including reactive oxygen species (ROS) and proteolytic enzymes, contribute to tissue damage and destruction.
    - Simultaneously, anti-inflammatory cytokines (e.g., interleukin-10) and pro-resolving mediators (e.g., lipoxins, resolving) are produced to dampen inflammation and promote tissue repair.

5. Resolution of Inflammation:

    - The inflammatory response is tightly regulated to prevent excessive tissue damage and promote resolution.
    - Pro-resolving mediators, such as specialized pro-resolving lipid mediators (SPMs), actively terminate inflammation by inhibiting pro-inflammatory signalling pathways and enhancing the clearance of apoptotic cells and debris.

6. Systemic Effects:

    - In addition to local tissue responses, inflammation can have systemic effects, including fever, leucocytosis, and acute-phase protein synthesis.
    - Systemic inflammatory responses may contribute to the pathogenesis of various diseases, including sepsis, autoimmune disorders, and cardiovascular diseases.

Understanding the dynamic interplay of cellular and molecular events underlying the inflammatory response provides insights into the pathophysiology of inflammatory diseases and informs the interpretation of inflammatory markers such as ESR. By elucidating the mechanisms of inflammation, researchers and clinicians can develop targeted therapeutic interventions to modulate the inflammatory response and improve patient outcomes in inflammatory conditions.

A. Interpretation of ESR results in clinical practice

Interpreting ESR results in clinical practice involves considering various factors, including the patient's medical history, clinical presentation, concurrent laboratory findings, and potential confounding factors. ESR is a nonspecific marker of inflammation and does not provide a definitive diagnosis but rather serves as a clue to the presence and severity of underlying inflammatory processes. Here is a breakdown of how ESR results are interpreted in clinical practice:

Normal Range:

- ESR values can vary depending on age, gender, and other demographic factors.
- In adults, the normal range for ESR is typically up to 20 mm/h in females and up to 15 mm/h in males.
- It's important to note that normal ESR values do not rule out the presence of inflammation, especially in cases of localized or mild inflammation.

Elevated ESR:

- Elevated ESR levels (>20 mm/h in females, >15 mm/h in males) are indicative of increased inflammation.
- The magnitude of ESR elevation may correlate with the severity and extent of inflammation, but it is not directly proportional.
- Elevated ESR can be seen in various inflammatory conditions, including infections, autoimmune diseases, malignancies, and tissue injury.

Clinical Correlation:

- Interpretation of ESR results should always be done in conjunction with the patient's clinical presentation and other laboratory findings.
- A thorough medical history, physical examination, and review of symptoms are essential for identifying potential underlying causes of inflammation.
- Additional diagnostic tests, such as imaging studies, microbiological cultures, serological assays, and tissue biopsies, may be necessary to confirm the diagnosis and guide management.

Differential Diagnosis:

- Elevated ESR is a nonspecific finding and does not provide information about the specific aetiology or pathogenesis of inflammation.
- A broad differential diagnosis should be considered, taking into account the patient's age, gender, comorbidities, and risk factors for various inflammatory conditions.
- Clinical judgment and expertise are required to prioritize diagnostic investigations and formulate a differential diagnosis based on the overall clinical context.

Monitoring Disease Activity:

- Serial measurements of ESR over time can provide valuable information about the course of inflammatory diseases and response to therapy.
- A decreasing trend in ESR levels may indicate a positive response to treatment, while persistently elevated ESR levels may suggest ongoing inflammation or treatment resistance.

However, it's essential to interpret changes in ESR values in conjunction with changes in clinical symptoms and other objective markers of disease activity.

In summary, interpreting ESR results in clinical practice requires a comprehensive approach that integrates clinical judgment, patient-specific factors, and relevant diagnostic information. ESR serves as a valuable adjunctive tool in the assessment of inflammation but should be interpreted cautiously in the context of the individual patient's clinical presentation and other laboratory findings.

B. Factors affecting ESR measurement

ESR measurement is influenced by various factors, both physiological and methodological, which can impact the accuracy and interpretation of results. Understanding these factors is crucial for clinicians to interpret ESR values correctly and make informed clinical decisions. Here's a deep dive into the factors affecting ESR measurement:

Physiological Factors:

a. Age and Gender: ESR values tend to be higher in females and increase with age. Hormonal fluctuations, such as those occurring during menstruation, pregnancy, or menopause, can also affect ESR levels.

b. Anaemia: ESR is inversely proportional to haematocrit and haemoglobin levels. Anaemia, whether due to nutritional deficiencies, chronic disease, or other causes, can lead to elevated ESR values.

c. Genetic Factors: Genetic variations may contribute to differences in ESR values among individuals, although specific genetic determinants have not been clearly elucidated.

Technical and Methodological Factors:

a. Sample Handling: Proper sample handling is essential to obtain accurate ESR measurements. Blood samples should be collected using standardized techniques, and anticoagulated promptly to prevent clotting. Inadequate mixing or agitation of samples can lead to inaccurate results.

b. Tube Size and Anticoagulant: The size and type of collection tubes (e.g., Westergren tubes, microhematocrit tubes) and anticoagulants used (e.g., sodium citrate, EDTA) can affect ESR measurements. Tubes with incorrect ratios of blood to anticoagulant or improper anticoagulant concentrations may yield inaccurate results.

c. Temperature and Time: ESR measurements are temperature-dependent, with higher temperatures leading to faster sedimentation rates. Standardization of incubation temperature (usually 20-25°C) and measurement time (typically 1 hour) is essential to ensure consistent and reproducible results.

d. Technical Variation: Variability in laboratory techniques, equipment calibration, and operator proficiency can contribute to inter-laboratory variability in ESR measurements. Regular quality control procedures and adherence to standardized protocols help minimize technical variation.

e. Red Blood Cell Aggregation: Factors that affect red blood cell aggregation, such as plasma viscosity, fibrinogen concentration, and protein composition, can influence ESR values. Conditions associated with increased plasma proteins or abnormal red blood cell morphology may lead to falsely elevated ESR results.

f. Inflammatory State: The presence of acute or chronic inflammation can significantly affect ESR values. Inflammatory cytokines, such as interleukin-6, stimulate hepatic synthesis of acute-phase proteins, including fibrinogen and C-reactive protein, which promote red blood cell aggregation and increase ESR.

g. Medications: Certain medications, such as corticosteroids, nonsteroidal anti-inflammatory drugs (NSAIDs), and oral contraceptives, can influence ESR measurements. Steroids may suppress inflammation and lower ESR, while NSAIDs and hormonal medications may have variable effects.

Other Factors:

a. Technical Artefacts: Presence of air bubbles, clots, or haemolysis in blood samples, as well as improper tube positioning during measurement, can lead to technical artefacts and inaccurate ESR readings.

b. Patient Positioning: Patient positioning during blood collection and measurement, such as tilting or shaking of tubes, can affect the distribution of red blood cells and influence ESR results.

In summary, ESR measurement is influenced by a multitude of factors, including physiological, technical, and methodological variables. Clinicians should be aware of these factors when interpreting ESR values and consider them in the context of the patient's clinical presentation and other laboratory findings to ensure accurate diagnosis and appropriate management of inflammatory conditions. Standardization of ESR measurement techniques, adherence to quality control procedures, and awareness of potential confounding factors are essential for reliable and reproducible ESR measurements in clinical practice.

C. Differential diagnosis based on ESR levels

Interpreting ESR levels in the context of differential diagnosis involves considering the patient's clinical presentation, medical history, and concurrent laboratory findings. While ESR is a nonspecific marker of inflammation, certain patterns of ESR elevation or depression can provide valuable clues to guide differential diagnosis. Here's a deep exploration of how ESR levels can inform the differential diagnosis:

1. **Elevated ESR:**
a) **Acute Inflammatory Conditions:**

- Infections: Bacterial, viral, fungal, or parasitic infections can lead to acute inflammation and elevated ESR. Conditions such as pneumonia, urinary tract infections, tuberculosis, and sepsis may present with markedly elevated ESR levels.
- Acute Rheumatic Fever: An autoimmune complication of untreated streptococcal pharyngitis, acute rheumatic fever is characterized by elevated ESR levels in conjunction with other clinical features such as migratory polyarthritis, carditis, and chorea.
- Acute Exacerbations of Chronic Inflammatory Diseases: Conditions such as rheumatoid arthritis, systemic lupus erythematosus, inflammatory bowel disease, and psoriatic arthritis may present with acute flares characterized by elevated ESR levels.

b. Chronic Inflammatory Conditions:

- Autoimmune Diseases: Systemic lupus erythematosus, rheumatoid arthritis, vasculitis, ankylosing spondylitis, and other autoimmune diseases are associated with chronic inflammation and persistently elevated ESR levels.
- Chronic Infections: Tuberculosis, osteomyelitis, chronic viral hepatitis, HIV/AIDS, and fungal infections may present with chronic inflammation and elevated ESR levels.
- Malignancies: Solid tumours (e.g., lung cancer, breast cancer, lymphoma) and hematologic malignancies (e.g., leukaemia, multiple myeloma) can induce chronic inflammation and elevate ESR levels.

c. Tissue Injury and Necrosis:

- Myocardial Infarction: Acute myocardial infarction and other forms of cardiac ischemia may lead to tissue injury and release of inflammatory cytokines, resulting in elevated ESR levels.
- Trauma and Surgery: Surgical procedures, traumatic injuries, burns, and tissue necrosis can induce acute-phase reactions and elevate ESR levels.

- Infarction and Embolism: Conditions such as pulmonary embolism, stroke, and mesenteric ischemia may cause tissue infarction and inflammation, leading to elevated ESR levels.

2. **Depressed ESR:**

a. Hyper viscosity Syndromes: Conditions associated with increased blood viscosity, such as polycythaemia vera, hyperglobulinemia, and hyperfibrinogenaemia, can impair red blood cell sedimentation and result in falsely depressed ESR levels.

b. Anaemia: Severe anaemia, particularly due to conditions such as sickle cell disease, thalassemia, or severe iron deficiency, can decrease red blood cell sedimentation and lead to decreased ESR levels.

c. Hypofibrinogenemia: Conditions associated with low fibrinogen levels, such as disseminated intravascular coagulation (DIC), liver failure, and certain congenital coagulation disorders, can result in decreased red blood cell aggregation and depressed ESR levels.

d. Technical Artefacts: Improper sample handling, air bubbles, clots, haemolysis, or technical errors during ESR measurement can lead to falsely depressed ESR values and should be considered in cases of unexpectedly low ESR levels.

In summary, differential diagnosis based on ESR levels involves considering the pattern and magnitude of ESR elevation or depression, along with the patient's clinical presentation and other laboratory findings. While elevated ESR is suggestive of inflammation and can aid in diagnosing various acute and chronic inflammatory conditions, depressed ESR may indicate underlying hyper viscosity syndromes, anaemia, hypofibrinogenemia, or technical artefacts. Clinicians should interpret ESR levels cautiously and integrate them into the broader clinical context to guide appropriate diagnostic evaluation and management decisions.

VII. Advances in ESR Measurement and Interpretation

Recent advances in technology and understanding have led to improvements in ESR measurement techniques and interpretation, enhancing the utility of this traditional inflammatory marker in clinical practice. This chapter explores the latest developments in ESR measurement and interpretation:

Automation and Standardization:

- Automated ESR analysers have replaced manual methods in many clinical laboratories, offering greater precision, reproducibility, and efficiency.
- These analysers utilize advanced optical or mechanical techniques to measure ESR directly from whole blood samples, minimizing pre-analytical variability and reducing turnaround time.

- Standardization efforts, such as the use of international reference materials and calibration standards, have helped harmonize ESR measurements across different laboratory platforms and minimize inter-laboratory variability.

High-Sensitivity ESR:

- High-sensitivity ESR methods, utilizing smaller blood volumes and shorter measurement times, have been developed to improve the detection of subtle changes in ESR levels, particularly in the low range.
- These methods may enhance the sensitivity of ESR as a marker of inflammation and enable earlier detection of disease activity or response to therapy in chronic inflammatory conditions.

Multimodal Inflammatory Markers:

- Integration of ESR with other inflammatory markers, such as C-reactive protein (CRP), serum amyloid A (SAA), and procalcitonin, provides a more comprehensive assessment of the inflammatory response.
- Combined measurement of ESR and CRP, for example, has been shown to improve diagnostic accuracy and prognostic value in various inflammatory diseases, including infections, autoimmune disorders, and malignancies.

Point-of-Care Testing:

- Advances in point-of-care testing technology have enabled rapid, near-patient measurement of ESR using handheld or desktop devices.
- Point-of-care ESR testing facilitates real-time monitoring of inflammation in outpatient settings, emergency departments, and ambulatory care settings, allowing for timely clinical decision-making and treatment optimization.

Molecular Insights into ESR Regulation:

- Emerging research has shed light on the molecular mechanisms underlying ESR regulation, providing insights into the factors influencing red blood cell aggregation and sedimentation.
- Understanding the interplay between inflammatory cytokines, red blood cell characteristics, and plasma factors may lead to novel therapeutic targets for modulating ESR and inflammation.

Personalized Interpretation:

- Advances in data analytics and machine learning algorithms hold promise for personalized interpretation of ESR results based on individual patient characteristics, clinical history, and biomarker profiles.
- Machine learning models trained on large datasets may help identify patterns and correlations in ESR data that predict disease outcomes, treatment response, or prognosis in specific patient populations.

In summary, advances in ESR measurement and interpretation have transformed this traditional inflammatory marker into a more sensitive, reliable, and clinically relevant tool for assessing inflammation in a variety of medical conditions. From automated analysers and high-sensitivity methods to multimodal inflammatory markers and point-of-care testing, these innovations have expanded the utility of ESR in clinical practice and paved the way for personalized approaches to inflammation assessment and management. Continued research and technological advancements in ESR measurement are expected to further enhance our understanding of inflammation and improve patient care in the years to come.

A. Modern techniques for ESR measurement

Modern techniques for ESR measurement have evolved significantly, offering improved accuracy, precision, and efficiency compared to traditional manual methods. These advancements have enhanced the utility of ESR as a marker of inflammation in clinical practice. Here, we delve deeply into the modern techniques for ESR measurement:

Automated ESR Analysers:

- Automated ESR analysers have largely replaced manual methods in clinical laboratories, offering several advantages, including:
- Precision: Automated analysers provide consistent and reproducible results, minimizing variability between measurements and operators.
- Efficiency: These analysers can process multiple samples simultaneously, reducing turnaround time and increasing laboratory throughput.
- Standardization: Automated systems are calibrated to international reference materials, ensuring standardization of ESR measurements across different laboratory platforms.
- Working Principle: Automated ESR analysers typically utilize advanced optical or mechanical techniques to measure erythrocyte sedimentation directly from whole blood samples. These methods often involve monitoring the rate of sedimentation in a closed system over a specified time period.

High-Sensitivity ESR Methods:

High-sensitivity ESR methods have been developed to improve the detection of subtle changes in ESR levels, particularly in the low range.

These methods utilize smaller blood volumes and shorter measurement times, allowing for more precise quantification of erythrocyte sedimentation.

High-sensitivity ESR techniques may enhance the sensitivity of ESR as a marker of inflammation, enabling earlier detection of disease activity or response to therapy in chronic inflammatory conditions.

Point-of-Care ESR Testing:

Point-of-care ESR testing has become increasingly available, allowing for rapid, near-patient measurement of ESR in various clinical settings.

Handheld or desktop devices enable real-time monitoring of inflammation, facilitating timely clinical decision-making and treatment optimization.

Point-of-care ESR testing is particularly valuable in outpatient settings, emergency departments, and ambulatory care settings where rapid assessment of inflammatory status is needed.

Multimodal Inflammatory Markers:

- Integration of ESR with other inflammatory markers, such as C-reactive protein (CRP) and serum amyloid A (SAA), provides a more comprehensive assessment of the inflammatory response.
- Combined measurement of ESR and CRP has been shown to improve diagnostic accuracy and prognostic value in various inflammatory diseases, including infections, autoimmune disorders, and malignancies.

Digital Health Solutions:

- Digital health solutions, including smartphone applications and web-based platforms, offer innovative approaches to ESR measurement and monitoring.
- These platforms may incorporate ESR measurements along with other clinical data, patient-reported outcomes, and biomarker profiles to provide personalized assessments of inflammatory status and disease activity.

In summary, modern techniques for ESR measurement have revolutionized the assessment of inflammation in clinical practice. From automated analysers and high-sensitivity methods to point-of-care testing and digital health solutions, these advancements have enhanced the accuracy, efficiency, and accessibility of ESR measurement, enabling more timely diagnosis and management of inflammatory conditions. Continued research and innovation in ESR measurement technologies are expected to further improve our understanding of inflammation and enhance patient care in the future.

B. Role of ESR kinetics in monitoring disease progression and treatment response

The kinetics of Erythrocyte Sedimentation Rate (ESR) play a crucial role in monitoring disease progression and evaluating treatment response in various medical conditions. Understanding the dynamic changes in ESR over time provides valuable insights into the course of inflammatory diseases and the effectiveness of therapeutic interventions. Here, we explore deeply the significance of ESR kinetics in clinical practice:

Disease Progression Monitoring:

- ESR kinetics are often used to track the progression of inflammatory diseases, such as rheumatoid arthritis, systemic lupus erythematosus, and inflammatory bowel disease.
- Rising ESR levels over time may indicate worsening inflammation and disease activity, prompting the need for intensification of treatment or modification of therapeutic regimens.
- Serial measurements of ESR allow clinicians to monitor the trajectory of disease progression and identify patients at higher risk of complications or poor outcomes.

Treatment Response Assessment:

- Changes in ESR levels following initiation of therapy serve as important indicators of treatment response and efficacy.
- Decreasing ESR levels over time suggest a favourable response to treatment, with reduction in inflammation and disease activity.
- Conversely, persistent elevation or fluctuation of ESR despite therapy may signal inadequate disease control, treatment resistance, or the need for alternative therapeutic strategies.
- Serial monitoring of ESR kinetics allows clinicians to assess the effectiveness of treatment interventions and adjust therapeutic regimens accordingly.

Prognostic Value:

- ESR kinetics provide prognostic information about disease outcomes and long-term prognosis.
- Rapid normalization of elevated ESR levels following treatment initiation may predict better clinical outcomes and reduced risk of disease relapse or progression.
- Conversely, persistently elevated or rising ESR levels despite treatment may portend poorer prognosis, increased risk of complications, or disease flares.

Timing of Measurements:

- The timing of ESR measurements is critical for accurately assessing disease progression and treatment response.
- Baseline ESR levels provide a reference point for comparison and help establish the severity of inflammation at the outset of treatment.
- Serial measurements at regular intervals, such as weekly, monthly, or quarterly, allow for tracking changes in ESR kinetics over time and evaluating the effectiveness of therapy.

Integration with Clinical Assessment:

- Interpretation of ESR kinetics should be integrated with clinical assessment, including patient-reported symptoms, physical examination findings, and other laboratory parameters.
- Clinicians should consider the overall clinical context when interpreting changes in ESR levels, taking into account factors such as concurrent medications, comorbidities, and lifestyle factors.

In summary, ESR kinetics serve as valuable biomarkers for monitoring disease progression and treatment response in inflammatory conditions. Serial measurements of ESR over time provide insights into the dynamic nature of inflammation, guiding clinical decision-making and optimizing therapeutic management. By incorporating ESR kinetics into routine clinical practice, clinicians can better assess disease activity, evaluate treatment efficacy, and improve patient outcomes in inflammatory diseases.

C. Future directions in ESR research

As technology advances and our understanding of inflammation deepens, the role of ESR continues to evolve. Future directions in ESR research hold promise for enhancing its clinical utility, elucidating underlying mechanisms, and exploring novel applications. Here's a deep exploration of the potential future directions in ESR research:

Mechanistic Insights:

- Further elucidation of the molecular mechanisms underlying ESR kinetics and regulation is essential for a comprehensive understanding of inflammation.
- Advances in molecular biology, genomics, and proteomics may uncover novel biomarkers and signalling pathways involved in erythrocyte sedimentation and aggregation.
- Understanding the interplay between inflammatory mediators, red blood cell characteristics, and plasma factors could lead to the identification of new therapeutic targets for modulating ESR and inflammation.

Personalized Medicine:

- Integration of ESR measurements with other clinical data, biomarkers, and imaging studies may enable personalized assessment and management of inflammatory conditions.
- Development of predictive models and algorithms using machine learning and artificial intelligence could facilitate risk stratification, treatment selection, and prognosis prediction based on individual patient characteristics and ESR kinetics.

Biomarker Discovery:

- Exploration of novel biomarkers associated with erythrocyte sedimentation and inflammation may expand our diagnostic and prognostic capabilities.
- Proteomic profiling, metabolomic analysis, and advanced imaging techniques may identify unique signatures and patterns associated with specific inflammatory diseases or treatment responses.
- Identification of biomarkers that correlate with ESR kinetics could enhance our ability to monitor disease progression, predict outcomes, and tailor therapeutic interventions.

Point-of-Care Technologies:

- Continued development of point-of-care ESR testing devices and platforms could improve accessibility and affordability of ESR measurement in resource-limited settings.
- Integration of ESR testing into portable diagnostic devices, wearable sensors, and telemedicine platforms may enable remote monitoring of inflammation and early detection of disease flares.
- Miniaturization of ESR measurement technology and incorporation into handheld devices could facilitate real-time monitoring of inflammatory status in ambulatory and home care settings.

Therapeutic Interventions:

- Exploration of novel therapeutic approaches targeting erythrocyte sedimentation and aggregation pathways may offer new avenues for the treatment of inflammatory diseases.
- Development of pharmacological agents, biologics, or gene therapies aimed at modulating ESR kinetics could complement existing anti-inflammatory treatments and improve patient outcomes.
- Clinical trials evaluating the efficacy and safety of novel ESR-modulating therapies in inflammatory conditions may pave the way for future therapeutic innovations.

Longitudinal Studies:

- Longitudinal cohort studies and clinical trials with extended follow-up periods are needed to better understand the long-term implications of ESR kinetics on disease progression, treatment response, and patient outcomes.
- Integration of ESR measurements into large-scale epidemiological studies and electronic health record databases could provide valuable insights into the epidemiology and natural history of inflammatory diseases.

In summary, future directions in ESR research hold great potential for advancing our understanding of inflammation, improving diagnostic and prognostic capabilities, and enhancing therapeutic interventions in inflammatory conditions. By harnessing technological innovations, biomarker discovery, personalized medicine approaches, and collaborative research efforts, we can unlock new insights into the role of ESR in health and disease, ultimately benefiting patient care and public health.

VIII. Clinical Implications and Future Perspectives

The clinical implications of Erythrocyte Sedimentation Rate (ESR) extend across various medical specialties, providing valuable insights into the diagnosis, monitoring, and management of inflammatory conditions. As we look to the future, there are several key clinical implications and future perspectives that warrant deep exploration:

Diagnostic Utility:

- ESR remains a widely used and valuable tool for diagnosing and assessing the severity of inflammation in a broad range of medical conditions.
- While ESR is nonspecific and cannot provide a definitive diagnosis, it serves as a complementary test alongside clinical evaluation and other laboratory investigations.
- Future research may focus on refining diagnostic algorithms and integrating ESR with other inflammatory markers to improve diagnostic accuracy and differentiate between different inflammatory diseases.

Monitoring Disease Activity:

- Serial measurements of ESR play a crucial role in monitoring disease activity, evaluating treatment response, and guiding therapeutic decisions in inflammatory conditions.
- ESR kinetics provide valuable insights into the dynamic nature of inflammation, allowing clinicians to track changes in disease progression over time and adjust treatment strategies accordingly.

- Future perspectives may involve the development of standardized protocols for serial ESR monitoring, incorporating digital health solutions for real-time data collection, and integrating ESR kinetics into clinical decision support systems.

Prognostic Value:

- ESR levels have prognostic implications for disease outcomes, treatment response, and long-term prognosis in inflammatory conditions.
- Elevated ESR levels are associated with increased morbidity, mortality, and disease complications, highlighting the importance of early identification and aggressive management of inflammation.
- Future research may explore novel biomarkers and imaging modalities to enhance prognostic prediction and risk stratification based on ESR kinetics and other clinical parameters.

Therapeutic Monitoring:

- ESR measurements are valuable for monitoring the efficacy and safety of therapeutic interventions in inflammatory diseases.
- Changes in ESR levels following treatment initiation or modification provide early indicators of treatment response and guide adjustments in therapy.
- Future perspectives may involve the development of targeted therapies aimed at modulating ESR kinetics and inflammation pathways, as well as the incorporation of ESR monitoring into personalized treatment algorithms.

Patient-Cantered Care:

- Incorporating patient-reported outcomes, preferences, and values into ESR monitoring and treatment decision-making is essential for patient-centred care.
- Clinicians should engage patients in shared decision-making, providing education, support, and empowerment to actively participate in their healthcare journey.
- Future perspectives may focus on enhancing patient engagement through digital health solutions, telemedicine platforms, and patient education materials tailored to individual needs.

Multidisciplinary Collaboration:

- Collaboration between healthcare providers, researchers, policymakers, and industry stakeholders is critical for advancing the clinical implications and future perspectives of ESR.
- Multidisciplinary teams can leverage expertise from different disciplines to address clinical challenges, design innovative research studies, and translate scientific discoveries into clinical practice.

- Future perspectives may involve fostering collaborative networks, promoting knowledge exchange, and facilitating interdisciplinary research initiatives to accelerate progress in ESR research and clinical applications.

In summary, Erythrocyte Sedimentation Rate (ESR) has profound clinical implications across various aspects of patient care, from diagnosis and monitoring to treatment and prognosis in inflammatory conditions. As we look to the future, integrating technological advancements, personalized medicine approaches, and patient-centred care principles will further enhance the clinical utility and impact of ESR in improving patient outcomes and advancing healthcare delivery.

A. ESR-guided management strategies in various diseases

ESR-guided management strategies play a significant role in the diagnosis, monitoring, and treatment of various diseases characterized by inflammation. By utilizing ESR as a biomarker, clinicians can tailor therapeutic interventions, monitor disease progression, and optimize patient outcomes. Here, we delve deeply into the application of ESR-guided management strategies across different medical conditions:

Inflammatory Joint Diseases:

- Rheumatoid Arthritis (RA): ESR is commonly used in the diagnosis and monitoring of RA. Elevated ESR levels correlate with disease activity and can guide treatment decisions, such as the initiation or adjustment of disease-modifying antirheumatic drugs (DMARDs) or biologic therapies.
- Osteoarthritis (OA): While ESR is generally within the normal range in OA, elevated levels may indicate concomitant inflammation or complications such as synovitis. ESR monitoring can help identify inflammatory OA subtypes and guide the use of anti-inflammatory medications or intra-articular injections.

Inflammatory Bowel Diseases (IBD):

Crohn's Disease and Ulcerative Colitis: ESR is used as a marker of disease activity and severity in IBD. Elevated ESR levels correlate with intestinal inflammation and can guide treatment decisions, such as the initiation or escalation of immunosuppressive therapies or biologic agents.

Infectious Diseases:

- Tuberculosis (TB): ESR is elevated in active TB and can aid in monitoring treatment response and identifying disease relapse. Serial ESR measurements are often used alongside microbiological tests to assess the effectiveness of anti-tuberculosis therapy.

- Pneumonia: Elevated ESR levels are commonly observed in bacterial pneumonia and can help differentiate bacterial from viral etiologist. Monitoring ESR kinetics can guide the duration of antibiotic therapy and assess treatment response.

Autoimmune Diseases:

- Systemic Lupus Erythematosus (SLE): ESR is a useful marker of disease activity and organ involvement in SLE. Elevated ESR levels may prompt further evaluation for lupus nephritis or other organ manifestations and guide treatment decisions.
- Multiple Sclerosis (MS): While ESR is not specific for MS, elevated levels may reflect systemic inflammation associated with disease activity. Monitoring ESR kinetics alongside clinical and radiological assessments can help guide treatment decisions in MS.

Cardiovascular Diseases:

- Acute Coronary Syndrome (ACS): Elevated ESR levels are associated with increased cardiovascular risk and adverse outcomes in ACS. ESR monitoring may help identify high-risk patients who may benefit from more aggressive management strategies or intensive secondary prevention measures.
- Atherosclerosis: Chronic low-grade inflammation plays a key role in the pathogenesis of atherosclerosis. Elevated ESR levels may indicate increased cardiovascular risk and guide risk stratification and preventive interventions.

Malignancies:

- Solid Tumours and Hematologic Malignancies: Elevated ESR levels are often observed in malignancies due to systemic inflammation or paraneoplastic syndromes. Monitoring ESR kinetics can provide valuable prognostic information and guide the evaluation of treatment response in cancer patients.

In summary, ESR-guided management strategies are employed across a spectrum of diseases characterized by inflammation, including inflammatory joint diseases, inflammatory bowel diseases, infectious diseases, autoimmune diseases, cardiovascular diseases, and malignancies. By integrating ESR monitoring into clinical practice, clinicians can optimize treatment decisions, monitor disease progression, and improve patient outcomes in various medical conditions. Continued research and innovation in ESR-guided management strategies hold promise for advancing personalized medicine and enhancing patient care in the future.

B. Potential role of ESR in personalized medicine

Personalized medicine aims to tailor medical treatment to individual patients based on their unique characteristics, including genetic makeup, environmental factors, and clinical presentation. ESR, as a widely used marker of inflammation, holds potential for integration into personalized medicine approaches across various medical conditions. Here, we delve deeply into the potential role of ESR in personalized medicine:

Disease Diagnosis and Subtyping:

- ESR can aid in the diagnosis and subtyping of inflammatory conditions by providing valuable information about the presence and severity of inflammation.
- In personalized medicine approaches, ESR measurements may complement other diagnostic tests and biomarkers to refine disease classification and guide therapeutic decisions.
- For example, in rheumatoid arthritis (RA), elevated ESR levels may indicate higher disease activity and help differentiate seropositive from seronegative subtypes, guiding the selection of targeted therapies.

Treatment Selection and Optimization:

- ESR-guided treatment strategies can help personalize therapeutic interventions based on individual patient characteristics and disease characteristics.
- Elevated ESR levels may indicate a more aggressive disease course or inadequate response to conventional therapies, prompting consideration of alternative treatment options.
- In diseases such as inflammatory bowel disease (IBD), ESR monitoring can guide the selection of immunosuppressive agents or biologic therapies tailored to disease severity and treatment response.

Monitoring Disease Activity and Treatment Response:

- Serial monitoring of ESR kinetics allows for dynamic assessment of disease activity and treatment response over time.
- In personalized medicine approaches, ESR measurements can be integrated with other clinical parameters, imaging studies, and biomarkers to optimize disease management and therapeutic decision-making.
- For example, in oncology, ESR kinetics may be used alongside tumour markers and imaging modalities to monitor tumour response to chemotherapy or immunotherapy and adjust treatment regimens accordingly.

Risk Stratification and Prognostication:

- ESR levels provide valuable prognostic information about disease outcomes, treatment response, and long-term prognosis.
- In personalized medicine approaches, ESR measurements can help stratify patients into risk categories based on their inflammatory status and predict disease progression or complications.
- For instance, in cardiovascular diseases, elevated ESR levels may indicate increased cardiovascular risk and prompt implementation of personalized preventive interventions, such as lifestyle modifications or pharmacological therapies.

Patient-Cantered Care and Shared Decision-Making:

- Incorporating ESR measurements into personalized medicine approaches promotes patient-centred care and shared decision-making.
- Clinicians can engage patients in discussions about their individual disease course, treatment options, and goals of care, taking into account ESR kinetics and other relevant clinical factors.
- By empowering patients to actively participate in their healthcare decisions, personalized medicine approaches incorporating ESR can improve treatment adherence, satisfaction, and overall patient outcomes.

In summary, Erythrocyte Sedimentation Rate (ESR) holds promise as a valuable biomarker in personalized medicine, offering insights into disease diagnosis, treatment selection, monitoring of disease activity and treatment response, risk stratification, and patient-centred care. By integrating ESR measurements into personalized medicine approaches, clinicians can optimize therapeutic strategies, improve patient outcomes, and advance precision medicine in various medical conditions. Continued research and clinical validation of ESR-guided personalized medicine approaches are essential for realizing the full potential of ESR in individualized patient care.

C. Emerging trends in inflammation research and implications for ESR

Inflammation research is a rapidly evolving field, driven by advances in technology, insights into molecular pathways, and a growing understanding of the role of inflammation in health and disease. These emerging trends have significant implications for the use of Erythrocyte Sedimentation Rate (ESR) as a biomarker of inflammation. Let's delve deeply into these emerging trends and their implications for ESR:

Molecular Mechanisms of Inflammation:

- Emerging research is elucidating the intricate molecular mechanisms underlying inflammation, including the role of cytokines, chemokines, and signalling pathways.
- Understanding these mechanisms may provide insights into the regulation of ESR kinetics and help identify novel biomarkers associated with specific inflammatory pathways.

- Implications for ESR: As our understanding of inflammation deepens, ESR may be used in conjunction with other inflammatory markers to characterize different inflammatory phenotypes and tailor treatment strategies accordingly.

Systems Biology Approaches:

- Systems biology approaches, such as genomics, transcriptomics, proteomics, and metabolomics, are revolutionizing our understanding of inflammation by analysing complex interactions within biological systems.
- Integration of multi-omics data may uncover new biomarkers and pathways associated with inflammation, providing a more comprehensive picture of inflammatory diseases.
- Implications for ESR: Integration of ESR measurements with multi-omics data could enhance our ability to stratify patients based on their inflammatory profiles and predict disease outcomes or treatment responses.

Immunometabolism and Metabolic Inflammation:

- The intersection of immunology and metabolism, known as immunometabolism, is a burgeoning area of research with implications for inflammatory diseases.
- Dysregulation of metabolic pathways can contribute to chronic low-grade inflammation, termed metabolic inflammation, and predispose individuals to metabolic disorders and cardiovascular diseases.
- Implications for ESR: ESR may serve as a marker of metabolic inflammation and cardiovascular risk, highlighting its utility beyond traditional inflammatory conditions and expanding its role in preventive medicine and chronic disease management.

Microbiome and Inflammation:

- The gut microbiome plays a critical role in modulating immune responses and inflammation, with implications for various inflammatory diseases, including inflammatory bowel disease, obesity, and autoimmune disorders.
- Alterations in gut microbiota composition, known as dysbiosis, can influence systemic inflammation and ESR levels through the production of microbial metabolites and activation of immune pathways.
- Implications for ESR: Monitoring ESR alongside assessment of gut microbiome composition may provide insights into the interplay between microbiota-host interactions and systemic inflammation, paving the way for personalized dietary or probiotic interventions.

Artificial Intelligence and Machine Learning:

- Artificial intelligence (AI) and machine learning algorithms are being increasingly utilized to analyse large-scale biological data and identify patterns associated with inflammation and disease.
- AI-driven approaches hold promise for predicting disease trajectories, identifying novel biomarkers, and optimizing treat mix. Conclusion Ent strategies through personalized predictive modelling.
- Implications for ESR: Integration of AI-based predictive models with ESR measurements may enhance risk stratification, prognosis prediction, and treatment selection in inflammatory diseases, enabling more precise and individualized patient care.

In summary, emerging trends in inflammation research offer exciting opportunities to deepen our understanding of the pathophysiology of inflammatory diseases and enhance the clinical utility of Erythrocyte Sedimentation Rate (ESR) as a biomarker. By leveraging insights from molecular mechanisms, systems biology approaches, immunometabolism, microbiome research, and artificial intelligence, we can harness the full potential of ESR to advance precision medicine and improve patient outcomes in inflammatory conditions. Continued interdisciplinary collaboration and translational research efforts are essential for translating these emerging trends into clinical practice and realizing the promise of personalized inflammatory medicine.

IX. Conclusion

In the conclusion of "ESR Unveiled: Understanding the Dynamics of Inflammation," we reflect on the significance of Erythrocyte Sedimentation Rate (ESR) as a biomarker of inflammation and its implications for clinical practice and research. Here, we summarize the key findings and insights gained from exploring the dynamics of inflammation through the lens of ESR:

Utility of ESR in Clinical Practice:

- ESR remains a valuable and widely used marker of inflammation, providing clinicians with valuable insights into the presence, severity, and course of inflammatory diseases.
- Through its simplicity, affordability, and widespread availability, ESR continues to play a crucial role in the diagnosis, monitoring, and management of various medical conditions across different specialties.

Evolution of ESR Measurement and Interpretation:

- Over the years, advancements in technology and understanding have transformed the measurement and interpretation of ESR, enhancing its accuracy, precision, and clinical relevance.
- From traditional manual methods to automated analysers and high-sensitivity techniques, ESR measurement has evolved to meet the demands of modern healthcare and personalized medicine.

Clinical Implications and Future Directions:

- ESR-guided management strategies offer personalized approaches to patient care, allowing clinicians to tailor treatment interventions based on individual patient characteristics and disease kinetics.
- Emerging trends in inflammation research, such as systems biology, immunometabolism, microbiome research, and artificial intelligence, hold promise for further advancing our understanding of inflammation and enhancing the clinical utility of ESR.

The Promise of Personalized Inflammatory Medicine:

- As we move towards a future of personalized medicine, ESR stands poised to play a central role in optimizing diagnostic and therapeutic strategies, improving patient outcomes, and advancing precision healthcare delivery.
- By integrating ESR measurements with other clinical data, biomarkers, and advanced analytical techniques, clinicians can gain deeper insights into the complex nature of inflammation and tailor interventions to meet the unique needs of individual patients.

In conclusion, "ESR Unveiled: Understanding the Dynamics of Inflammation" underscores the enduring importance of Erythrocyte Sedimentation Rate (ESR) as a cornerstone in the assessment of inflammation. Through comprehensive exploration and deep understanding, we have unveiled the dynamics of inflammation and its implications for clinical practice and research. As we continue to advance our knowledge and capabilities, ESR remains a vital tool in the arsenal of healthcare providers, guiding decisions and improving outcomes in the management of inflammatory diseases.

Printed in Dunstable, United Kingdom